THE

MET
FLEX
DIET

ALSO BY IAN K. SMITH, M.D.

NONFICTION

Plant Power

Burn Melt Shred

Fast Burn

Mind over Weight

Clean & Lean

The Clean 20

Blast the Sugar Out!

The SHRED Power Cleanse

The SHRED Diet Cookbook

SUPER SHRED

SHRED

The Truth About Men

Eat

Happy

The 4 Day Diet

Extreme Fat Smash Diet

The Fat Smash Diet

The Take-Control Diet

Dr. Ian Smith's Guide to Medical Websites

FICTION

Wolf Point

The Unspoken

The Ancient Nine

The Blackbird Papers

THE

MET
FLEX
DIET

BURN BETTER FUEL,
BURN MORE FAT

IAN K. SMITH, M.D.

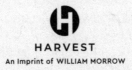

HARVEST
An Imprint of WILLIAM MORROW

This book contains advice and information relating to health care. It should be used to supplement rather than replace the advice of your doctor or another trained health professional. If you know or suspect you have a health problem, it is recommended that you seek your physician's advice before embarking on any medical program or treatment. All efforts have been made to ensure the accuracy of the information contained in this book as of the date of publication. This publisher and the author disclaim liability for any medical outcomes that may occur as a result of applying the methods suggested in this book.

FIRST EDITION

Designed by Renata DiBiase
Illustrations on pages 241 and 244 by Alexis Seabrook

Library of Congress Cataloging-in-Publication Data has been applied for.

ISBN 978-0-06-328982-6

23 24 25 26 27 LBC 5 4 3 2 1

To my mother, Rena, who is always willing to try my new programs and who is always honest in her assessments, as mothers tend to be. I'm forever grateful for all of your sacrifices and support and, most important, for teaching me how to fight.

CONTENTS

A NOTE FROM
THE AUTHOR

I've been researching, studying, and writing about nutrition, health, and fitness for a long time. I've personally corresponded with tens of thousands of people looking to improve their diet and fitness levels and lose weight. In many respects, I feel like I've seen and heard it all; however, I'm absolutely certain there's still a lot out there for me to learn, and this presents an infinite number of opportunities to grow intellectually and expand my knowledge base. These yet-to-be-discovered opportunities excite and fuel my desire to keep exploring and creating as I work to help others find answers to health challenges they so desperately want or need.

As much as I've tried to understand new scientific concepts and principles, I've always strived to understand the concerns and feedback of everyday people who are hungry to make positive changes so they can lead healthier, more satisfying lives. However, there are some things that have stumped me along the way. One of those things has been the assortment of statements I've heard from many people over the years in reference to carbs. "I can just look at carbs and gain weight." "Carbs and I simply don't get along." "The second I eat carbs my body starts gaining weight." Maybe you too have made one of these statements or share the sentiments they convey. Well, you're not alone, and honestly, I never fully grasped the underpinnings of these statements—until *now*!

Months before I decided to write this book, I came across a term I had never heard before—"metabolic flexibility." It looked and sounded scientifically cool, and I was excited to read about it to see what it meant. After very quickly learning the definition and physiologic underpinning of this term, I thought about those carb statements I'd been hearing for years but never fully understood. Metabolic flexibility addresses the body's ability (or inability) to switch from burning carbs to burning fats and vice versa. I had one of those eureka moments as the last twist of the bulb finally turned on the light in my brain. What all of these people (and I'm sure millions of others) have been feeling and describing is a state of metabolic inflexibility. It isn't necessarily that the carbs themselves are bad, but rather that their bodies have a difficult time processing them effectively and efficiently. That's why they feel the way they do when eating carbs.

When you put the wrong oil in a car's engine or the engine isn't given proper care and maintenance, its performance level starts to diminish, and you eventually begin to feel this operational decline while driving the car. If the problem or problems aren't corrected before too much damage is done, the engine simply dies, and you have a huge, costly problem on your hands. Well, millions of people are driving a car (their body) whose engine (their metabolism) is sputtering and triggering warning lights that are either going unrecognized or being purposely ignored. **The Met Flex Diet** is a program that will tune up your engine so you can not only lose weight but also operate at peak performance to hold off disease and cover hundreds of thousands of miles of open road before it's time for a check-in with the mechanic. In fact, with this six-week program, you become your own mechanic and wrestle with your destiny so that it falls back under your control—exactly where it should be.

Ian K. Smith, M.D.
April 2023

1

WHAT IS METABOLIC FLEXIBILITY?

To understand the concept of metabolic flexibility, you first must understand the concept of metabolism. There's no doubt in my mind that everyone reading this book has heard the word "metabolism"; however, many of you might not understand exactly what it means and what its full array of implications are for your health. So let's get a basic understanding of this critical physiologic concept that can have a tremendous impact not just on that number you see on the scale but on how you actually look and feel.

METABOLISM

If asked what the word "metabolism" means, most people would say, "How fast my body can burn calories." That basic understanding still holds true. However, your metabolism isn't some magical thing inside of your body that just chews up calories, nor is it an organ, like the heart, lungs, or liver. Rather, your metabolism is the collective effort of billions of cells in your body that are carrying out chemical processes (work) every second of your life—even when you're sleeping—that allow you to live and function and be who you are. Just as a lawn mower requires fuel or a battery to operate and a washing machine needs some type of power source to turn on and spin, the billions of cells that make up your body require energy to do all of the amazing things they do. These chemical processes make up what we call a person's metabolism, and they can be quite complicated. Your cells need energy to do what they do, and one of the ways they get their energy is by converting the food you eat into energy. Just as height is measured in feet and inches, energy also has a way of being measured, in what we call calories. When you read on the back of a yogurt container that it contains 150 calories, what you're being told is that the yogurt is storing 150 units of energy (calories) that your body can use after it breaks the food down in your digestive system.

Your metabolism is constantly working. Throughout the day it operates at different intensity levels. It's active when you're sleeping, but not as active as when you're walking or climbing steps or taking a shower. It's active even when you are in a deep sleep and your body is at rest, because you still need energy to power the activities that keep you alive: your heart is still beating, your lungs are still breathing, and your blood is still circulating throughout your body. Your metabolism provides you with energy for small functions, such as sending neurologic messages from your brain to the rest of your body, as well as large functions, such as digesting food, keeping your body temperature in a normal range, and many other processes that occur every second of every day of your life.

Metabolism can be separated into two major branches of activities—catabolism and anabolism. Catabolism is typically defined as a process of breaking down. A series of reactions occur that take relatively large molecules and break them down into smaller ones. During this breakdown, energy is released that the cells in your body can use to carry out their functions. A critical catabolic process in the body is digestion. When you eat food, your body needs to break it down into small, simple nutrients that can be used to fuel your daily activities of living.

Anabolism, the second and equally important branch of your metabolism, is exactly the opposite of catabolism. Anabolic processes take smaller units, like the amino acids from food, and bind them together to create larger structures called protein. In other words, your body takes the energy that is released through catabolism and uses it to build relatively large, complex molecules.

A term most people have heard and are typically concerned about is "metabolic rate." This is the rate at which your body burns energy in a certain period. When people say they have a "fast metabolism," they're typically referring to the metabolic rate, which, as you now know, is just part of the entire metabolism picture. Metabolic rate determines how fast your body can use, or "burn," the calories that come from food. If you have a slow metabolic rate, then it would follow that you don't burn through the calories from that piece of cake as quickly as other people with a faster metabolic rate. You are more likely to gain weight because, if you have energy you can't use, then your body has to do something with it, and that means storing it in the form of fat.

Understanding our metabolism has been a key concept in trying to understand the rates at which we gain weight and why two people of similar weight, musculature, height, and other characteristics can eat the same number of calories per day and have the same level of physical activity, yet one of them gains weight faster than the other. We have always pointed to the difference in their metabolism or metabolic rate as a central explanation for the difference in weight gain—or in some cases weight loss—between them.

The conventional wisdom has always held that as we age our metabolism slows down—specifically that around the age of 30 our metabolic rate really begins to take a nosedive, then continues slowing down every year. This continual metabolic rate decline has been highlighted as the major contributing factor to the weight gain many experience as they get older. It's also been widely accepted that as women near menopause their metabolism slows dramatically. What we have long believed to be indisputable facts about metabolism, however, have actually been largely refuted by a major paper titled "Daily Energy Expenditure through the Human Life Course," published in the journal *Science* in August 2021. Among the many findings reported in the paper, one of the most significant is that metabolism has four distinct life stages and differs for all people across these stages.

The Four Stages of Metabolism

1. Infancy up until age 1: Calorie burning is at its peak and accelerates until it's 50 percent above the adult rate.

2. From age 1 until around age 20: Metabolism gradually slows by approximately 3 percent a year.

3. Ages 20 to 60: Metabolism holds relatively stable.

4. After age 60: Metabolism declines about 0.7 percent a year.

These researchers also found that despite what many have advocated and believed over the years, there really aren't any differences in metabolism between men and women when we control for body size and the amount of muscle people have. They also note that these findings apply to the general population, but of course there are individual cases that can be regarded as exceptions to the rules. Some people have metabolic rates that are about 25 percent below the average for their age, while others have a rate that can be 25 percent above average. Regardless, metabolism for the vast majority of people tends to be within a certain range, thus throwing a huge bucket of water on the belief that metabolism alone is the difference in why people gain and lose weight at different rates.

Despite this new evidence suggesting that there are no wide differences in metabolic rates for most of the population, there's also important evidence that we can alter our metabolic rate. Although this rate alteration might not be permanent, there are ways to make it go high enough for a long enough period of time to make a difference in how we burn or use food calories and store fat. Think about driving your car down a highway and setting it on cruise control. Your car will do whatever it needs based on the road conditions to keep the car moving at the speed that you've set. When you're going uphill, your car will work harder to keep the pace, and conversely, your car will back the engine off and allow gravity to do more of the work of keeping the pace going downhill. When you press the gas pedal, the car will go faster than the cruise speed you set. It will stay at the higher speed as long as you're pressing the pedal, but when you stop pressing, the vehicle will gradually slow down and then reengage the set cruise control speed. Your metabolism works the same way. Like most people, you have a genetically determined metabolic rate that is like your cruise control speed that keeps you motoring along. There are things you can do, however, that will temporarily boost your metabolic rate—the equivalent of pressing the gas pedal to make your car go faster. The good news is that while you don't have control of your genetically determined metabolic rate, you do have control over some of these metabolic boosters.

Metabolic Boosters

- Increase protein consumption
- Work out with high-intensity interval training (HIIT)

- Build more lean muscles
- Drink more water
- Snack often
- Increase B12 consumption

Although metabolism is still not fully understood, its implications for how we gain and lose weight and its impact on our overall health have never been more important in our need to prevent and identify causes for various conditions. The National Center for Advancing Translational Sciences currently recognizes more than 500 metabolic disorders, albeit many of them are rare. The health of our metabolism is just one factor in the more global concept of our overall metabolic health. The prevailing definition of metabolic health is having ideal levels of blood sugar, triglycerides, high-density lipoprotein (HDL) cholesterol, blood pressure, and waist circumference, without using medications. Why do these specific factors matter? Researchers have shown that they directly relate to our risk for diabetes, heart disease, and stroke. In fact, a 2019 seminal study on metabolic health published by researchers from the University of North Carolina at Chapel Hill found that only 12 percent (one out of eight) of US adults have optimal metabolic health.[1] This obviously does not paint a flattering picture of where we stand with regard to metabolic health, but where there's a challenge, there's also tremendous opportunity. The Met Flex Diet program has been constructed to help you create and take advantage of this opportunity.

METABOLIC FLEXIBILITY

The "Met Flex" in the title of this book stands for "metabolic flexibility." Simply defined, metabolic flexibility is the ability of the body's cells to effectively switch between the fuel sources they use to power their activities. The two major fuel sources for the body are carbohydrates and fats. You're considered metabolically flexible when you can burn either fuel efficiently when it's available. An analogy that might explain this better is that between a hybrid car and a traditional gasoline-powered car. A hybrid electric car has both a battery and a fuel tank. The car can be operated on battery power, but when the battery is almost depleted, it switches to gas from the fuel tank as its energy source. A hybrid car represents the metabolically flexible state, because it can use whatever power source is available. A gasoline-powered car, however, can only use gas as its power source. Unfortunately, once the gas tank is empty, the car can no longer run until more fuel is pumped into it. A car with no ability to switch and use another power source would be considered metabolically inflexible.

Our bodies typically prefer to burn fuel in the form of the food we consume, which is broken down in our digestive tract into basic nutrients such as carbohydrates (glucose), fat, and protein. We eat food, digest it, extract energy from it, and then carry out our daily functions of living. What happens when we have depleted all of the energy from the food we've eaten and we don't eat again for a while? Our body still needs energy to function, even if we're just lying in bed. Our heart is still pumping, and our lungs are still expanding and contracting to bring vital oxygen into our bodies. We need to find other fuel sources once our food energy is gone, so the body turns to plan B—burning fat. The often-dreaded fat is not something we want around our organs (visceral fat) or underneath our skin (subcutaneous fat) not only because we may not like how we look but also because it can have detrimental effects on our health. However, fat is a stored form of energy, and when the body no longer has its preferred energy source (food) available, it turns to fat, breaks it down (catabolism), and converts it into energy units that can be used. Fat becomes our fuel source when nothing else is available, and without it we would die. We are metabolically flexible when we can burn food nutrients when they're available and use our stored fat as our fuel when they're not.

ENERGY EXTRACTION FROM FOOD

This is how the body extracts energy from food after eating. The body stores this energy in our liver and muscle in the form of glycogen when we don't burn enough of it and there's some left over.

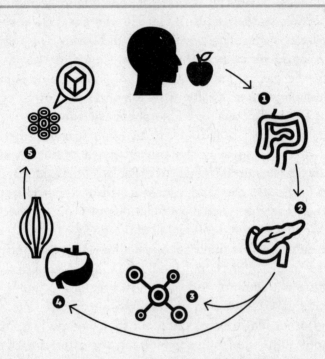

1. Food broken down by digestive system into glucose to be used as energy.

2. Pancreas secretes the hormone insulin into the bloodstream to help transport glucose into the cells throughout the body.

3. Insulin helps glucose from the blood to be transported into cells where it's used as energy.

4. Insulin facilitates glucose being stored in the liver and skeletal muscle in the form of glycogen.

5. Excess glucose is stored as fat to be used later when energy is needed.

FAT BURNING DURING FASTING

During the fasting state, glycogen stores in the liver and muscle are broken down and glucose is released into the blood. Once these stores are depleted, the body switches to using fat. Fatty acids are taken up by the liver and used to form ketone bodies, which are then the energy used by cells.

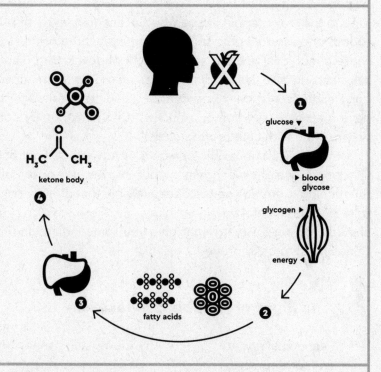

1. The liver and skeletal muscle are prompted to break down their glycogen stores and release glucose into the blood to be used for energy.

2. Fat cells are prompted to break down and release fatty acids into the blood.

3. Fatty acids taken up by the liver are converted to ketone bodies (ketosis), which are then released into the blood.

4. Ketone bodies are absorbed by the cells throughout the body, where they are now the new fuel source instead of glucose.

No blood test is currently available to test a person's metabolic flexibility. However, empirical data and the abundance of certain medical conditions suggest that a large number of people are metabolically inflexible. One of the biggest concerns is something called metabolic syndrome, which is the presence of three or more of five conditions: high blood pressure, high blood glucose (sugar) levels, high levels of triglycerides (a type of fat) in the blood, a large circumference around the waist (apple-shaped body), and low levels of HDL (good) cholesterol in the blood. If you have three or more of these conditions, you are at higher risk of developing diabetes, heart disease, and stroke. In fact, according to the American Heart Association, 23 percent of US adults are thought to have metabolic syndrome, a number that is extremely concerning to health care professionals.

A metabolically inflexible person is disadvantaged not only in terms of weight management but in other areas of daily functioning. Currently no tests are available that directly compute or assess metabolic inflexibility, but there are signs you should look out for that might give you some indication that things need to be improved.

Signs of Metabolic Inflexibility

- Feelings of anxiety and/or depression
- A need for some type of stimulant like coffee to function
- Difficulty losing fat
- Constant cravings despite recently eating
- Fatigue, sluggishness, or crankiness when not eating (fasting)
- Fatigue after a carbohydrate-rich meal like pasta
- Fluctuating blood sugar levels

BENEFITS OF
METABOLIC FLEXIBILITY

Just as a runner can improve their time running the mile and a weightlifter can improve how many times they can lift a 50-pound dumbbell, you can improve your body's ability to switch from burning one fuel to another. You can also improve how efficiently your body burns these fuels. Awaiting you once this happens are many potential benefits, some of which are listed here. Keep these benefits in mind as you go through the Met Flex Diet program so that, if you feel challenged at some point, you can remind yourself of all the reasons why you started in the first place.

Benefits of Improved
Metabolic Flexibility

- Improved weight loss and better weight management
- Improved blood sugar level control
- Increased energy levels
- Better sleep
- Better overall health
- Decreased risk of developing metabolic disease (like metabolic syndrome)
- Reduced cravings

2

IMPROVING YOUR METABOLIC FLEXIBILITY

Now that you understand the concept of metabolic flexibility and its critical impact on your weight and overall health, it's time to learn what you can do right now to begin improving it. There's a tremendous amount of ongoing research trying to determine the best strategies for enhancing metabolic flexibility. In the meantime, researchers have identified several areas of change that can help you achieve this improvement.

Ways to Improve Metabolic Flexibility

- Exercise
- Intermittent fasting
- Cyclical ketosis
- Better sleep hygiene
- Dietary pattern shift

EXERCISE

That there are benefits of exercise to overall good health is nothing groundbreaking. Everyone knows that being physically active and not sedentary has major implications for weight loss, the cardiovascular system, muscles, joints, and various other areas of the body. It is also well-known that regular physical activity or exercise is important to prevent and manage several diseases such as high blood pressure, type 2 diabetes, heart disease, and stroke. Exercise, particularly the type of exercise you do, can also be extremely effective at improving your metabolic flexibility.

For the sake of simplicity, let's divide exercise into three groups: cardiovascular exercise (aerobic exercise like walking or jumping rope), resistance training (weight lifting and resistance bands), and high-intensity interval training (HIIT, intervals of intense exertion alternating with intervals of rest or low exertion). Each type of exercise affects the body in a different way, especially in relation to how we consume energy (burn calories). During the course of my six-week plan, you will be asked to perform all three types of exercise at different times. This is part of my plan because when it comes to improving metabolic flexibility, not all exercise is created equal.

Several studies, including one published in the *American Journal of Physiology: Endocrinology and Metabolism* and one in the *Journal of Physiology*, have examined the direct impact of exercise on metabolic flexibility, and the results have been tremendously instructive.[1] According to the American Diabetes Association, physical activity can lower blood sugar levels up to 24 hours or more after a workout because exercise makes the body more sensitive to the actions of the insulin hormone. One of these studies compared obese and lean individuals who were given a high-fat diet over a three-day period.[2] The lean individuals responded by increasing the fat burn rate in their muscles; the obese individuals were not able to generate a similar response, thus signaling impaired metabolic flexibility. After ten consecutive days of aerobic activity, however, this impairment was no longer observed. The obese individuals adapted and were able to increase their fat burn rate just as the leaner individuals did.

Scientists and exercise physiologists have worked tirelessly to answer the million-dollar question: What kind of exercise is best for fat burning? Intuitively, we think that the harder we work out and the more we sweat and become fatigued, the more fat we burn. Research results have indicated, however, that this is not necessarily the case. In fact, optimal fat burning occurs during lower-intensity exercise, not when we're exercising so vigorously that we're about to drop from exhaustion.

Understanding the extreme benefits of exercise in improving metabolic flexibility requires first understanding that exercise significantly increases the body's demand for energy and that the two major energy sources to supply this power are carbohydrates and fat. Sometimes both sources are used at the same time, and often one is used more than the other. The basic premise of the crossover concept—an important concept in exercise and fuel usage defined many years ago by the researchers George Austin Brooks and Jacques Mercier—is that at lower intensities of exercise fats are the primary source of energy. As the exercise intensity increases, fats are used less and carbohydrates are used more. As the exercise intensity continues to increase there comes a point when carbs and fats are used equally to fuel the body. As exercise increases beyond this point, however, carbs are used more and fat usage decreases. The point at which that change occurs is called the crossover.

Exercise physiologists have divided exercise into fat-burning and cardio zones. The fat-burning zone typically refers to low-intensity aerobic activity that keeps your heart rate between 60 and 69 percent of your maximum heart rate (maximum heart rate = 220 – your age). When your body is in this zone, you are burning a higher percentage of calories from fat. The cardio zone refers to high-intensity aerobic activity that keeps your heart rate between 70 and 85 percent of your maximum heart rate. In the cardio zone, carbs are the predominant fuel burned, but a significant amount of fat is still being burned. However, when you consider which level of exercise burns the most overall calories, there's no doubt that high-intensity activity wins the battle, underscoring the importance of varying the type and duration of your exercise to achieve your weight loss and metabolic goals. The exercise portion of the Met Flex Diet plan you're about to follow incorporates this variety.

Doing strength or resistance training is an anaerobic exercise. That means it doesn't require oxygen. In fact, it almost exclusively burns carbohydrates stored in the muscles for energy. Unlike cardio, this type of exercise is performed at maximal effort for a short period of time, using quick bursts of energy. Building more lean muscle mass increases your metabolic rate because muscle tissue burns more calories than fat. This is why, when you're trying to lose weight, it's important not to ignore the need to improve or maintain some degree of lean muscle mass. Beyond weight loss, improving the strength of your muscles has other benefits, including joint protection, increased bone strength and density, and reduction of the risk of diabetes and heart disease.

HIIT exercises will also be part of your exercise regimen, and for good reason. Not only does this workout, conducted in episodic bursts, burn an increased number of calories during your training session, but calories will continue to be burned throughout the day long after you stop exercising, owing to a concept called excess post-exercise oxygen consumption (EPOC). According to this concept, the higher the exercise intensity, the more your body is stressed, and thus the more energy and oxygen your body needs to repair and recover once the workout is over. HIIT is performed by alternating between periods of high-intensity exercise and periods of rest or low-intensity exercise. You will find out more about this exercise method in chapter 11.

All three categories of exercise do their part in helping you maintain maximal metabolic flexibility. Cardio improves how well the microscopic mitochondria in your cells work, which is important because the mitochondria are responsible for the production of adenosine triphosphate (ATP), a critical factor in producing energy. Strength training will help make your cells more sensitive to the insulin hormone. Increasing insulin sensitivity can be important in helping your cells take glucose out of the blood, thus improving your blood sugar level management. HIIT exercises burn lots of carbs, but they can also burn fat once the carb sources are depleted. The long recovery from HIIT gives your body more time to keep burning calories.

INTERMITTENT FASTING

You've probably heard of the term "intermittent fasting," or IF. This eating style is exactly what it sounds like—periods of fasting alternating with periods of eating. There are many versions of IF, but the three major types are the 5:2 method, time-restricted feeding (TRF), and alternate-day fasting. These methods use different strategies, but all three strive to achieve the same results and share the basic method of alternating between regulated periods of eating and fasting periods. Alternation can be advantageous to achieving metabolic flexibility because it is teaching your body how to survive in different food and energy environments based on what's available at any given time.

In the 5:2 method, you are instructed to eat in your typical fashion for five days of the week, then restrict yourself to consuming no more than 500 calories during the other two days. These two "fasting" days are not allowed to be consecutive.

The time-restricted feeding method is the most commonly and widely used. The 24-hour day is divided into two periods, eating and fasting, which are referred to as an "eating window" and a "fasting window." You consume all of your meals during the eating window and eat no food at all during the fasting window, though you can consume beverages as long as they don't add up to more than 50 calories collectively.

Alternate-day fasting calls for normal eating one day followed by a day of relative fasting when you consume no more than 500 calories. The key to this method's success is rigidly sticking to the limited calorie count on the fasting days, even though you are allowed to eat whatever you want on the eating day. In most versions of this method, you are allowed to drink as many calorie-free beverages as you want on the fasting day. This is helpful considering there are so few calories allowed and liquids can help you achieve some level of satiety faster and more easily. During the six-week **Met Flex Diet** meal plan, you will be following a combination of these different IF methods.

While scientists continue to study and clarify why intermittent fasting is so beneficial to metabolism and cellular health, there is a working hypothesis that much of it has to do with the fasting phase of the strategy. During the fasting phase, researchers surmise, cells are subjected to mild stress and are in a fight to survive. The cells are willing to do whatever it takes to live, so they make adaptations that improve their ability to handle the stress they experience during the fasting phase. These are the adaptations that scientist believe make the cells more resilient and better equipped at both preventing and, if necessary, fighting disease.

Another mechanism by which fasting can be beneficial to our cells is described by a concept called "autophagy." As many as 30 to 40 trillion microscopic cells are constantly at work throughout the body to make us who we are and help us do what we want to do. Let's compare what happens to our cells to what happens to our cars. Driving your car on long trips in heavy traffic every day is stressful to the mechanical operation of your vehicle. Over time your car begins to wear down, and certain parts, having become less functional, need to be repaired or replaced. You take your car to the mechanic, who performs a service by replacing parts or fixing the old ones so that they operate better. By the same token, as we get on with our lives—standing up in the morning, sitting on a train going to work, walking around a grocery store—our cells experience general wear and tear. Infections, inflammation, and other medical conditions add to the stress on our cells, which causes damage to the tiny but important parts inside of the cells called organelles. Our bodies have an amazing system whereby we serve as our own repairmen. These damaged components are inspected and salvaged where possible, but if the damage is too great, they are completely broken down, degraded, and recycled. This recycled material can then be used either to create new cells or to serve as an energy source for those other cells. All of this happens in our bodies every second of every day, and we are not even aware that it's going on. When you are fasting, you are starving the cells, causing stress that triggers the process of autophagy, which leads to digesting the cell parts and providing critical energy for cellular survival.

Research has suggested that intermittent fasting offers a variety of benefits, many of them having nothing to do with weight loss. While the primary concern of the Met Flex Diet plan is metabolic flexibility and weight loss, there's absolutely nothing wrong with receiving the additional perks that come with this style of eating.

In this program, we are going to try a combination of the IF strategies. You might find that one or two are easier for you, and that's to be expected. Do your best, however, to follow all of the eating regimens as instructed, as the timing of meals and your fasting can be just as critical as what you eat and the number of calories you consume.

Intermittent Fasting Benefits

- Weight loss
- Decreased inflammation
- Reduced insulin resistance
- Decreased belly fat
- Preserved learning and memory functioning
- Improvement in asthma-related symptoms

CYCLICAL KETOSIS

I have never been a supporter of keto diets, despite the overwhelming evidence that in the short term this style of eating can be effective at helping with weight loss. My opposition has been based not on the results that many have achieved but rather on the types of food, particularly the amount of fat, that people must eat on keto to find success. The vast preponderance of research over the last few decades has demonstrated that high-fat, overly high-protein diets can pose a serious risk to your health, particularly the cardiovascular system and the kidneys. A substantial amount of conflicting research, however, has kept this area of study murky. Some studies, including one published in the journal *Nutrients*, have actually suggested that very low-carb diets (keto) actually lower the risk of heart disease and help people suffering from metabolic syndrome, insulin resistance, and type 2 diabetes, at least in the short term.[3] Research is expanding to examine whether keto has a positive impact on other medical conditions, such as acne, nervous system diseases, and cancer. This lack of clear and convincing evidence has led to the wide disagreements among health care professionals about the benefits and dangers of keto.

Ketosis is the process that occurs when your body doesn't have enough carbohydrates (glucose) to burn as a source of fuel. Since its carbohydrate supply is depleted, the body must find another source. Luckily, we have fat, which can be burned to make molecules called ketones, and ketones can be used by the body as a fuel source when no carbohydrates are available. The keto diet essentially starves your body of carbohydrates, thus forcing your body to turn to your stored fat as well as the fat you consume in your food as fuel sources. This is why people tend to lose weight and fat on a keto diet.

A typical ketogenic diet stresses high fat consumption with very few carbs, typically not more than 50 grams of carbs per day. A cyclical ketogenic diet is a variant of the standard keto.

It is a regimen that basically forces you in and out of ketosis by having you follow a standard ketogenic diet for five or six days per week, followed by one or two days of higher carb consumption. The idea is simple: you are putting yourself into ketosis on the days when your fat intake is high and your carb intake is extremely low. You then spend one or two days eating lots of carbs to allow your body to adjust to burning carbs again now that they are available. The belief is that alternating between carb availability and fat availability teaches your body how to become more metabolically flexible by learning how to adapt and burn whatever fuel is available.

The **Met Flex Diet** plan will introduce cyclical ketosis for the last four weeks. During that period, it will be critical that you stay mindful of what you eat and the relative ratio of nutrients. For the keto part of the week, you should expect to consume as much as 70 to 90 percent of your daily calorie intake in the form of fatty foods. The key to success, however, will be to choose the healthier fats—monounsaturated and polyunsaturated. You will try to limit your consumption of saturated fats, while totally avoiding the dreaded trans fats.

Sources of Healthy Fats

- Avocados
- Eggs
- Extra-virgin olive oil
- Fatty fish (anchovies, herring, mackerel, salmon, sardines, trout, and tuna)
- Flaxseed
- Full-fat dairy products (like cheese and yogurt)
- Nut butters
- Nuts and seeds (almonds, walnuts, Brazil nuts, chia seeds, hemp seeds, sunflower seeds)
- Olives
- Tofu
- Yogurt (full-fat)

The next macronutrient to consider is protein, which should comprise approximately 10 to 20 percent of your total calories. Every cell in the human body contains proteins, which are involved in almost all bodily functions and processes. Proteins are composed of smaller units called amino acids, and together they make up our body's tissues, the enzymes that are important for chemical reactions to occur, and the transporters that carry atoms and small molecules within the cells and throughout the body. There has been some debate about how much protein we need to consume on a daily basis. The National Academy of Medicine recommends that adults consume a minimum of 0.8 grams of protein for every kilogram of body weight per day. For those who see the world in pounds, that's slightly over 7 grams for every 20 pounds of body weight. Thus, a 140-pound person should consume 50 grams of protein each day, and a 200-pound person should consume 70 grams.

There will be plenty of protein options on the Met Flex Diet plan, but it's important to keep in mind that reducing your consumption of processed meats (bacon, hot dogs, sausages, and cold cuts) is important for your overall health. According to the Nutrition Source from the Harvard School of Public Health, processed meats are those that have been "transformed through salting, curing, fermentation, smoking, or other processes to enhance flavor or improve preservation."[4]

Common Sources of Protein

- Dairy (cheese, yogurt, milk)
- Eggs
- Fish (including shellfish)
- Legumes (beans and lentils)
- Nuts
- Poultry (chicken, duck, turkey)
- Red meat (beef, goat, lamb, pork, veal)
- Seeds
- Soy

Carbohydrates will reenter your eating regimen during the first two days of the week. Eating carbs will break the ketosis phase that you have been in for the previous five days and allow your body to switch from burning fat to burning carbs. On these two carb-loading days, as much as 60 to 70 percent of your calories will come from carbs, 15 to 20 percent of your calories will come from protein, and only 5 to 10 percent of your total calories will come from fat. Notice that these percentages are completely opposite to what is expected during the five-day ketosis period of the week. These two days can be optimized by focusing on eating more complex carbs rather than simple carbs. Complex carbs are more nutritious, tend to be higher in fiber, and are digested more slowly. Fiber and starch are considered complex carbs.

Examples of Complex Carbs

- Asparagus
- Barley
- Beans
- Broccoli
- Brown rice
- Buckwheat
- Carrots
- Chickpeas
- Cucumbers
- Fruits (strawberries, apples, grapefruit, pears, prunes)
- Green beans
- Lentils
- Oatmeal
- Onions
- Peas
- Potatoes
- Quinoa
- Spinach
- Sweet potatoes
- Wheat
- 100 percent whole-wheat bread
- Zucchini

Simple carbs are like fast-burning fuels that quickly break down into sugars after we eat them. They include glucose, fructose, sucrose, table sugar, raw sugar, brown sugar, corn syrup, and high-fructose corn syrup. Simple carbs cause our blood sugar level to rise quickly because they are broken down in our body at such a rapid pace. It's best to reduce your consumption of simple carbs, or even avoid them altogether, as much as possible.

Although there is great flexibility in the food choices on the **Met Flex Diet** plan, it's important that you follow the timing of food consumption and exercise as closely as possible. I have carefully combined several strategies to yield maximal results. It's often the case that what and when you eat relative to when you exercise and the type of exercise you do makes a difference in the fuel your body uses and thus in improving your metabolic flexibility results. Nothing in this plan is gratuitous. It's all part of a bigger strategy that, when followed closely, will give you the highest likelihood of success in increasing your metabolic flexibility. Believe in yourself. Believe in the plan. Embrace the process as you go forward!

3

WEEK 1
FUNDAMENTAL

Welcome to the first week of improving your metabolic flexibility and teaching your body how to adapt to whatever food environment you might encounter. This first week is all about setting the stage for the rest of the program so that you'll find the most success possible. The plan for these pivotal seven days has been constructed in a way that allows you to jump right into the program and start seeing results quickly and consistently.

The best way to attack this plan is to be prepared, so it's important to sit down for a few minutes and take a look at what's in the daily meal plans for the week. You should preselect your meal and snack choices for the week so that you can create a shopping list that ensures that you stock the foods that will help you achieve the greatest compliance with the plan and, ultimately, success in using it. Not having the right foods, or not having enough of them, can tempt you to improvise, and before you know it you've strayed far from the plan. This is where trouble can start. There's a reason for everything planned not just for this week but for all six weeks, so don't dismiss any detail as trivial or irrelevant to the overall mission. Don't forget: you are trying this plan most likely because whatever you've done in the past hasn't been successful or you haven't been able to maintain success. So do your best to follow the plan as written. That said, by no means do I expect you to follow it perfectly, as no one is perfect. But give it your best effort and make good choices as often as you can.

For the next six weeks you will have plenty of food and beverage options. When you are in the keto portion of the diet, it's important to closely follow what is suggested, because eating or drinking too many carbs will break your state of ketosis and prevent your body from reaching the ultimate goal of burning the fat you eat (dietary) and the fat stored in your body. The two tables here provide a general guideline to the types of cheese you can eat and to some of the foods, ingredients, and beverages you should avoid. It's virtually impossible to list everything, so I assembled a list that covers most of the important categories. Always refer to the specific guidelines for a particular week to get a better handle on what is permitted. The guidelines at the beginning of each week change, but the guidelines in these tables are consistent throughout the plan.

Cheeses Allowed

- Blue cheese
- Brie
- Camembert
- Cheddar
- Colby jack
- Cottage cheese
- Cream cheese
- Feta
- Goat cheese (chèvre)
- Halloumi
- Havarti
- Limburger
- Manchego
- Mascarpone
- Mozzarella
- Muenster
- Parmesan
- Pepper jack
- Provolone
- Romano
- String cheese
- Swiss cheese

FOOD, INGREDIENTS, AND BEVERAGES TO AVOID ON KETO DAYS

BEVERAGES

ALCOHOL	Beer (regular), Bloody Mary, Cosmopolitan, Margarita, Piña Colada, Rum and Coke, Sangria, Whiskey Sour, White Russian
ALCOHOLIC COOLERS	Alcopops, spirit coolers, wine coolers, hard lemonades
DRINKS	Sugary drinks (soda, fruit juice, punch, lemonade, sweet teas)

FOOD

FRUIT	All, except limited amounts of blueberries, strawberries, blackberries, and raspberries
GRAINS/ STARCHES	Bread, wheat-based products, rice, pasta, cereal
SWEET TREATS	Cakes, cookies, doughnuts, pastries, candy, regular ice cream, Italian ice (keto ice cream is allowed)
VEGETABLES	Potatoes (white and sweet), parsnips, carrots, rutabagas, corn, leeks, beets
BEANS OR OTHER LEGUMES	Black beans, peas, kidney beans, lentils, chickpeas
CONDIMENTS	Barbecue sauce, honey mustard, teriyaki sauce, ketchup

GUIDELINES

Here are your guidelines for this week. You are going to be following the time-restricted feeding method of intermittent fasting, so that is the most important part of making this week a success.

- **Eating Schedule.** You will have 10 hours to consume all of your food and beverages with calories (eating window). The next 14 hours are going to be your fasting window. During your fast you can have as many no-calorie beverages as you like, but if you do want to have some beverages like coffee or tea during this period, make sure the calories you drink don't total more than 50 calories. The timing of your eating and fasting windows is completely up to you and your schedule, but here's a sample of what a 14:10 day might look like.

FEEDING WINDOW	FASTING WINDOW
10:00 AM–8:00 PM	8:00 PM–10:00 AM

- **Water.** You must consume one cup of water before each meal. You can drink more water during and after the meal, but one cup must be consumed before your first bite.

- **Fruits and Vegetables.** They can be frozen or fresh. You can have canned, but that is the last option, as they tend to be packed with lots of salt and other preservatives. If possible, consume only vegetables and fruits with no added ingredients. If eating canned, make sure it is low-sodium (140 milligrams or less per serving).

- **Alcohol.** You're allowed to drink alcohol this week, but remember, you're trying to lose weight and improve your metabolic flexibility. Too much alcohol is going to make it that much more difficult to reach your goals. You are allowed to drink only low-carb alcohol. You can consume alcohol on the following days—days 1, 2, 3, 4, 5, 6, and 7. You are allowed only one drink on those days, either a "lite" beer or a mixed drink. The table here lists the allowed alcoholic beverages and mixers and their quantities.

TYPE OF ALCOHOL	SERVING SIZE ALLOWED
Gin	1.5 ounces (44 milliliters)
"Lite" beer	12 ounces (355 milliliters)
Red wine	5 ounces (148 milliliters)
Tequila	1.5 ounces (44 milliliters)
Vodka	1.5 ounces (44 milliliters)
Whiskey	1.5 ounces (44 milliliters)
White wine	5 ounces (148 milliliters)

TYPE OF MIXER	SERVING SIZE ALLOWED
Diet soda	½ cup
Seltzer	Unrestricted
Sugar-free tonic water	Unrestricted

- **Soda.** Neither regular nor diet soda is allowed. This is very important. If you're someone who drinks sodas, please try to eliminate them from your diet. If you can't, at least cut your consumption in half. The one exception is diet soda as a mixer in your alcoholic beverage (see the alcohol guidelines table).

- **Sugar.** No table or cane sugar is allowed, but you can have sweeteners like organic stevia, organic monk fruit, pure or raw honey, yacón syrup, or organic erythritol. (Be careful not to consume too much erythritol as it can cause diarrhea.)

- **Syrup.** You are allowed to use sugar-free or no-added-sugar syrups. If you can find organic syrup, then all the better.

- **Coffee.** You can have coffee during your fasting periods, but you can't load it up with calories. During your fasting period you can't consume more than 50 calories total, and adding cream and sugar to your coffee could take you over that mark. On your keto (low-carb) days, be mindful of what you put in your coffee, as you can't consume more than 50 grams of carbs for the entire day. Some coffee preparations have so many carbs that you could drink your entire day's allowance, and then some, in a single cup.

- **Meal Swaps.** Sometimes the plan might present you with meal options that you don't like, or that have ingredients you don't have access to. Don't panic. You are allowed to swap meals as long as you swap them in the same category (breakfast, lunch, dinner, meal 1, meal 2) and on the same type of day (carb-loading, 500 calories or less, and so on).

- **Ingredient Elimination.** If a meal option includes an ingredient or food that you don't like, have an allergy to, or simply don't have access to, feel free to eliminate it and just use the rest of the ingredients and foods.

- **Snacks.** Please try to consume only the snacks that are listed in the daily meal plan or in chapter 10. If for some reason you need to eat a snack that's not listed, make sure it's no more than 150 calories.

- **Exercise.** The exercise is written specifically to complement the fasting method as well as the meal plan. Pay close attention to the instructions. You can find examples of the exercises in chapter 11.

DAY 1
BREAKFAST

Choose one of the following:

- 2 pancakes with 2 slices of bacon (beef or pork) and ½ cup fruit
- 2 scrambled eggs with cheese and diced vegetables

LUNCH

Choose one of the following:

- Large green salad: 3 cups greens of your choice with sliced peaches, goat cheese, cucumbers, almonds, basil, and 2 to 3 tablespoons balsamic vinaigrette
- Turkey, chicken, ham, or tuna salad sandwich on the bread of your choice with lettuce, tomato, a slice of cheese, and 1 teaspoon of your preferred condiment

THE SLEEPY ADVANTAGE

A good night's rest is more than just what your parents insisted you get on a school night. Abundant, restful sleep is important for our bodies to function at peak performance. Many people have busy lives and experience various stressors that use up an inordinate amount of time and mental energy. However, sleep is not a luxury even in a busy life or for someone with a demanding job. In fact, just the opposite is true. Sleep is a necessity.

The body has four biological categories of rhythms, which are determined by genetics. One of these categories is circadian rhythms: the 24-hour cycle connected to day and night that serves as part of the body's internal clock running in the background to ensure that the body's functions and processes are optimized at various points during every 24-hour period. The sleep-wake cycle is one of these rhythms. Severe or frequent disruptions to the rhythm of this cycle can affect many things, such as the body's natural flow of hormones, with real physiologic consequences for our functioning and our overall health. It has been well documented in medical literature that a lack of sleep can increase levels of the hormone ghrelin (hunger) and decrease levels of the hormone leptin (satiety). This is how a lack of sleep can lead to increased hunger and appetite.

The bottom line: if you want to lose weight and increase your metabolic flexibility, turn off the electronics and get some good shut-eye.

DINNER

Choose one of the following:

- 6 ounces grilled or baked chicken breast (skinless) with 1 medium baked potato (optional additions: ½ teaspoon butter or sour cream, chives, broccoli, and cheese)
- 6 ounces grilled or baked fish of your choice with 2 vegetables of your choice

SNACKS

Each day choose two from the following list to consume anytime of the day (but not consecutively and not within an hour before or after eating a meal):

- ½ small apple, sliced, with 2 teaspoons peanut butter
- ¼ cup loosely packed raisins
- Kale chips: ⅔ cup raw kale, stems removed, baked with 1 teaspoon extra-virgin olive oil at 400°F until crisp
- ½ medium baked potato with 1 teaspoon butter or 1 tablespoon sour cream
- ½ cup low-fat or fat-free plain Greek yogurt with a dash of cinnamon and 1 teaspoon honey

EXERCISE

AM OR PM

Twenty minutes of strength training (see chapter 11 for exercise examples). Consume at least 20 grams of protein and 15 grams of carbs within an hour of finishing your workout.

DAY 2

BREAKFAST

Choose one of the following:

- 1 cup cooked oatmeal with ¼ cup fruit (optional additions: 1 teaspoon brown sugar, 1 pat of butter, ¼ cup milk)
- Grilled cheese sandwich made with 2 slices of 100 percent whole-grain or whole-wheat bread (3.5 inches by 3.5 inches) and 2 ounces cheese

LUNCH

Choose one of the following:

- Tuna salad sandwich (2 ice cream scoops' worth) on the bread of your choice (optional addition: lettuce)
- 6-ounce beef or turkey burger on a bun of your choice stacked with cheese, lettuce, and tomato, with a small green garden salad

DINNER

Choose one of the following:

- 1 serving of vegetable or meat lasagna (2 inches by 4 inches by 3 inches) and a small green garden salad
- 6 ounces fish (grilled or baked) with 2 servings of vegetables

SNACKS

Choose two of the following to consume anytime of the day (but not consecutively and not within an hour before or after eating a meal):

- Leaf lettuce roll-up stuffed with a single slice of ham or beef and cabbage, carrots, or peppers
- Tropical cottage cheese: ½ cup fat-free cottage cheese with ½ cup chopped fresh mango and pineapple
- 6 large clams
- 3 ounces cooked fresh crab
- 15 mini pretzel sticks with 2 tablespoons fat-free cream cheese

EXERCISE

AM

Twenty-minute "fasted workout" (don't eat beforehand) and lower-intensity cardio exercise (see chapter 11 for exercise examples). Besides not eating anything before your workout, do not eat for at least two hours after.

PM

Twenty-minute HIIT session. Don't eat anything for at least an hour afterward (see chapter 11 for exercise examples).

DAY 3
BREAKFAST

Choose one of the following:

- 12-ounce smoothie (see chapter 9 for recipes)
- 8-ounce Greek yogurt parfait with granola

LUNCH

Choose one of the following:

- Spaghetti and meatballs (2 cups cooked pasta and 2 meatballs) in a tomato-based sauce
- Chicken sandwich with tomato, cheese, lettuce, and 1 tablespoon of your preferred condiment, on the bread of your choice, and a small green garden salad with 1 tablespoon dressing

DINNER

Choose one of the following:

- 3 to 4 servings of vegetables and 1 cup brown rice
- 1½ cups chicken or beef stir-fry with 1 cup brown rice

SNACKS

Choose two of the following to consume anytime of the day (but not consecutively and not within an hour before or after eating a meal):

- 1 cup mixed berries (raspberries, blueberries, or blackberries)
- Citrus-berry salad: 1 cup mixed berries (raspberries, strawberries, blueberries, and blackberries) tossed with 1 tablespoon freshly squeezed orange juice
- 1 medium red pepper, sliced, with 2 tablespoons soft goat cheese
- 10 baby carrots with 2 tablespoons hummus

- 1 small scoop (the size of 2 golf balls) of low-fat frozen yogurt

EXERCISE

Rest day. If you still want to exercise, do a low-intensity cardio workout for 15 to 20 minutes. This will be a bonus workout, and it will help you achieve your goals faster (see chapter 11 for exercise examples).

DAY 4
BREAKFAST

Choose one of the following:

- 2 cups (or less) of cold cereal (no sugar) with the milk of your choice and 1 piece of fruit
- 2-egg omelet and chopped vegetables of your choice

LUNCH

Choose one of the following:

- Large salad with 3 cups greens of your choice and 2 to 3 tablespoons dressing of your choice (optional additions: mushrooms, beets, cucumbers, rice, sunflower seeds, and basil)
- 2 slices of cheese, pepperoni, or veggie pizza (5 inches wide by 6 inches long)

DINNER

Choose one of the following:

- 2 cups cooked whole-wheat pasta, 3 ounces diced chicken, and vegetables of your choice
- 6 ounces grilled fish, chicken, or steak, with 2 servings of vegetables of your choice

SNACKS

Choose two of the following to consume anytime of the day (but not consecutively and not within an hour before or after eating a meal):

- Leaf lettuce roll-up stuffed with a single slice of ham or beef and cabbage, carrots, or peppers
- Tropical cottage cheese: ½ cup fat-free cottage cheese with ½ cup chopped fresh mango and pineapple
- 6 large clams
- 3 ounces cooked fresh crab
- 15 mini pretzel sticks with 2 tablespoons fat-free cream cheese

EXERCISE

AM

Twenty-minute fasted workout and lower-intensity cardio exercise (see chapter 11 for exercise examples). Don't eat anything before your workout and for at least two hours after.

PM

Fifteen-minute lower-intensity cardio workout. Don't eat anything for at least an hour after (see chapter 11 for exercise examples).

DAY 5

BREAKFAST

Choose one of the following:

- One 8-inch waffle or two 4-inch waffles with 2 slices of bacon (pork or turkey), 2 link sausages (3 inches long), or 1 sausage patty (3 inches wide) (optional additions: butter and syrup)
- Egg-white omelet made with whites of 2 eggs and diced vegetables

LUNCH

Choose one of the following:

- 1 large chili dog (no bun) and a small green garden salad
- Bacon cheeseburger (no bun) and a small green garden salad

DINNER

Choose one of the following:

- 3 small beef, chicken, or fish tacos
- 2 pieces of fried chicken and a serving of leafy green vegetables

SNACKS

Choose two of the following to consume anytime of the day (but not consecutively and not within an hour before or after eating a meal):

- 1 hard-boiled egg with "everything" bagel seasoning

- 8 to 10 chocolate kisses
- 1½ ounces cooked Pacific halibut
- 2 ounces cooked lobster
- 25 oyster crackers

EXERCISE

AM OR PM

Twenty minutes of strength training (see chapter 11 for exercise examples). Consume at least 20 grams of protein and 15 grams of carbs within an hour of finishing your workout.

DAY 6
BREAKFAST

Choose one of the following:

- ½ cup fruit and 2 slices of bacon (pork or turkey)
- 12-ounce smoothie (see chapter 9 for recipes)

LUNCH

Choose one of the following:

- Large salad with 2 cups spinach or kale, 3 ounces chicken, onions, broccoli, shredded cabbage, brown, white, or wild rice, basil, and 2 to 3 tablespoons teriyaki-based dressing or another dressing of your choice
- 6 ounces grilled salmon, mackerel, trout, whitefish, or fried catfish and a small green garden salad

DINNER

Choose one of the following:

- 2 cups beef, chicken, turkey, or fish stew
- 6 pieces sushi of your choice (avocado rolls, cucumber and avocado rolls, shrimp tempura rolls, spicy tuna rolls, or California rolls)

SNACKS

Choose two of the following to consume anytime of the day (but not consecutively and not within an hour before or after eating a meal):

- 2 medium kiwis
- ¼ avocado, smashed, on a whole-grain cracker, sprinkled with balsamic vinegar and sea salt
- 5 cucumber slices topped with ⅓ cup cottage cheese and salt and pepper
- White bean salad: ⅓ cup white beans, a squeeze of lemon juice, ¼ cup diced tomato, and 4 cucumber slices
- 2 strips of low-fat string cheese

EXERCISE

AM

Twenty-minute fasted workout and lower-intensity cardio exercise (see chapter 11 for exercise examples). Don't eat anything before your workout and for at least two hours after.

DAY 7
BREAKFAST

Choose one of the following:

- 1 slice of avocado toast: mash 1 small avocado in a bowl, then spread on 1 slice of 100 percent whole-grain or whole-wheat toast (optional additions: sea salt and tomato)
- Bacon, egg, and cheese sandwich on toast or English muffin

LUNCH

Choose one of the following:

- 1 cup soup, such as minestrone, chicken noodle, vegetable, bean, tomato, squash, lentil, or split pea (but no potatoes or cream), with a small green garden salad
- 5-ounce turkey, chicken, salmon, or veggie burger on a bun of your choice (optional additions: 1 slice of cheese, tomato, and lettuce)

DINNER

Choose one of the following:

- 1 serving of lasagna (meat or meatless, 2 inches by 4 inches by 3 inches), with a small green garden salad
- 2 cups cooked spaghetti and three 2-inch meatballs with a small green garden salad

SNACKS

Choose two of the following to consume anytime of the day (but not consecutively and not within an hour before or after eating a meal):

- ½ cup fat-free yogurt and ½ cup blueberries
- ½ whole-wheat English muffin topped with 1 teaspoon fruit butter
- 4 cooked large sea scallops
- 2 ounces cooked yellowfin tuna

EXERCISE

Rest day. If you still want to exercise, do a low-intensity cardio workout for 15 to 20 minutes. This will be a bonus workout, and it will help you achieve your goals faster (see chapter 11 for exercise examples).

4

WEEK 2
ADAPTATION

This week is all about pushing your body to make the necessary adaptations to a new way of eating and moving. Since this is only your second week, your body is still making adjustments, not only to the food you're eating but also to your new exercise regimen. Do your best to stick to the plan and keep believing that even if you aren't seeing the results yet, they are coming.

This week we are going to employ the 5:2 method of fasting. This is very different from last week's time-restricted feeding, so you need to read through the week's meal plan and be prepared. Remember, having two fasting days doesn't mean you can go crazy and eat anything you want, in whatever quantity you want, on the five nonfasting days. Please be mindful of the timeless axiom that calorie counts still matter and calories in should be less than calories out to achieve optimal weight loss. Choose wisely on those five days and make sure you do your exercise, which is especially important when you are consuming a lot more calories than you will during the fasting days.

GUIDELINES

Here are your guidelines for this week. You are going to be following the 5:2 method of intermittent fasting, so be mindful of and prepared for the fasting days. The low-calorie days are spaced apart so that you won't be struggling through consecutive fasting days.

- **Eating Schedule.** You will have five days of relatively normal eating and two days of low-calorie eating (fasting). Don't switch the days in the program, as they are in a particular order for good reason. On your fasting days, I strongly encourage you not to eat on the run, but rather to take the time to sit down in a relaxed setting and to eat and savor your food.

- **Water.** You must consume one cup of water before each meal. You can drink more water during and after the meal, but one cup must be consumed before your first bite.

- **Fruits and Vegetables.** They can be frozen or fresh. You can have canned, but that is the last option, as they tend to be packed with lots of salt and other preservatives. If possible, eat only vegetables and fruits with no added ingredients. If eating canned, make sure it is low-sodium (140 milligrams or less per serving).

- **Alcohol.** You're allowed to drink alcohol this week, but remember, you're trying to lose weight and improve your metabolic flexibility. Too much alcohol is going to make it that much more difficult to reach your goals. You are allowed to drink only low-carb alcohol. You can consume alcohol on the following days—days 1, 2, 4, 6, and 7. You are allowed only one drink on those days, either a "lite beer" or a mixed drink. The table here lists the allowed alcoholic beverages and mixers and their quantities.

TYPE OF ALCOHOL	SERVING SIZE ALLOWED
Gin	1.5 ounces (44 milliliters)
"Lite" beer	12 ounces (355 milliliters)
Red wine	5 ounces (148 milliliters)
Tequila	1.5 ounces (44 milliliters)
Vodka	1.5 ounces (44 milliliters)
Whiskey	1.5 ounces (44 milliliters)
White wine	5 ounces (148 milliliters)

TYPE OF MIXER	SERVING SIZE ALLOWED
Diet soda	½ cup
Seltzer	Unrestricted
Sugar-free tonic water	Unrestricted

- **Soda.** Neither regular nor diet soda is allowed. This is very important. If you're someone who drinks sodas, please try to eliminate them from your diet, but if you can't, at least cut your consumption in half. The one exception is diet soda as a mixer in your alcoholic beverage (see the alcohol guidelines table).

- **Sugar.** No table or cane sugar is allowed, but you can have sweeteners like organic stevia, organic monk fruit, pure or raw honey, or organic erythritol. (Be careful not to consume too much erythritol as it can cause diarrhea.)

- **Syrup.** You are allowed to use sugar-free or no-added-sugar syrups. If you can find organic syrup, then all the better.

- **Coffee.** You can have coffee during your fasting periods, but you can't load it up with calories. During your fasting period you can't consume more than 50 calories total, and adding cream and sugar to your coffee could take you over that mark. On your keto (low-carb) days, be mindful of what you put in your coffee, as you can't consume more than 50 grams of carbs for the entire day. Some coffee preparations have so many carbs that you could drink your entire day's allowance, and then some, in a single cup.

- **Meal Swaps.** Sometimes the plan might present you with meal options that you don't like, or that have ingredients you don't have access to. Don't panic. You are allowed to swap meals as long as you swap them in the same category (breakfast, lunch, dinner, meal 1, meal 2) and on the same type of day (carb-loading, 500 calories or less, and so on).

- **Ingredient Elimination.** If there's an ingredient or food that you don't like, have an allergy to, or simply don't have access to, feel free to eliminate it and just use the rest of the ingredients and foods.

- **Snacks.** Please try to consume only the snacks that are listed in the daily meal plan or in chapter 10. If for some reason you need to eat a snack that's not listed, make sure it's no more than 150 calories. On the two fasting days, you will be allowed to have one snack from those that are listed, so choose wisely, as it will be critical in helping you stretch your calories throughout the day as much as possible.

- **Exercise.** The exercise is written specifically to complement the fasting method as well as the meal plan. Pay close attention to the instructions. You can find examples of the exercises in chapter 11.

DAY 1
BREAKFAST

Choose one of the following:

- Fruit plate or fruit salad with 6-ounce yogurt
- Egg frittata made with 2 eggs, cheese, and your choice of vegetables

LUNCH

Choose one of the following:

- 1½ cups chicken or beef stir-fry
- Large salad with 2 cups greens of your choice, roasted sweet potato wedges, shaved Parmesan, raw beets, broccoli, tomatoes, basil, and 2 to 3 tablespoons balsamic vinaigrette or dressing of your choice

DINNER

Choose one of the following:

- Vegetarian plate: 3 to 4 servings of cooked vegetables (1 serving is about ½ cup cooked vegetables)
- 2 cups cooked pasta (white or whole-wheat) with 3 ounces diced chicken or fish and tomatoes, broccoli, or vegetable of your choice

HIIT IS A BIG HIT

High-intensity interval training has a number of advantages compared to traditional steady-state workouts. This energy-burst training style not only does wonders for your heart health but has an important impact on your metabolic flexibility, specifically on your body's ability to switch to burning fat. The creators of Lumen, the metabolism tracker company, examined data from over 1 million pre- and post-workout metabolic measurements and found that 60 percent of HIIT workouts resulted in shifting the body from carb burn to fat burn. This was a significant increase from the shift to fat burn found among 50 percent of participants whose daily exercise was running and cycling.

So how much HIIT should you do during the week? In the absence of a universal standard, the US Department of Health and Human Services recommends doing this type of vigorous exercise two to three times per week for 30 to 45 minutes per session. As impactful as HIIT exercises can be, be aware of the possibility of getting too much of a good thing. Too much HIIT can actually hinder your metabolism, something you obviously don't want to happen. Like most things in life, moderation is the key when it comes to HIIT workouts.

SNACKS

Choose two of the following to consume anytime of the day (but not consecutively and not within an hour before or after eating a meal):

- Stuffed figs: 2 small, dried figs stuffed with 1 tablespoon reduced-fat ricotta and sprinkled with cinnamon
- 1 cup cherries
- ⅓ cup wasabi peas
- ½ cucumber (seeded) stuffed with one thin slice of lean turkey and mustard or fat-free mayonnaise
- 10 to 16 cashews

EXERCISE

AM

Twenty-minute fasted workout and lower-intensity cardio exercise (see chapter 11 for exercise examples). Don't eat anything for at least two hours after the workout.

DAY 2
BREAKFAST

Choose one of the following:

- Protein shake (350 calories or less)
- Fruit smoothie (350 calories or less)

LUNCH

Choose one of the following:

- 1½ cups pasta with sun-dried tomatoes or other vegetables in a noncreamy sauce
- Large salad with 3 cups greens of your choice and 2 to 3 tablespoons dressing of your choice (optional additions: mushrooms, beets, cucumbers, rice, sunflower seeds, and basil)

DINNER

Choose one of the following:

- Chicken Broccoli Casserole (page 169)
- 1 cup lentil soup with a small green garden salad

SNACKS

Choose two of the following to consume anytime of the day (but not consecutively and not within an hour before or after eating a meal):

- ½ cup low-fat cottage cheese with ¼ cup fresh pineapple slices
- ½ cup low-fat cottage cheese mixed with 1 tablespoon natural peanut butter
- 2 slices of deli turkey breast
- Watermelon salad: 1 cup raw spinach with ⅔ cup diced watermelon, sprinkled with 1 tablespoon balsamic vinegar
- 8 small shrimp and 3 tablespoons cocktail sauce

EXERCISE

AM

Twenty-minute fasted workout, lower-intensity cardio exercises, and 15 minutes of strength training (see chapter 11 for exercise examples). Don't eat anything before the workout and for at least two hours after the workout.

DAY 3

500-CALORIE FASTING DAY

You must consume six to ten cups of no-calorie water today. This is critical. Try squeezing a little fresh lemon juice into your water to help suppress your appetite longer. You will eat only two meals and one snack during this day, so make sure you space them properly as they need to stretch the entire day. Your calorie intake will be very low today, so adjust your physical activity accordingly. The goal is to train your body to mobilize your fat stores to be used for energy.

MEAL 1

Choose one of the following:

- 1½ cups soup, such as tomato, cucumber, chicken, squash, black bean, white bean, lentil, or turkey, and a small green garden salad with 1 tablespoon dressing
- 12-ounce smoothie (200 calories or less)
- 1 scrambled egg and 1 slice of bacon

MEAL 2

Choose one of the following:

- 4-ounce turkey burger (no bun)
- 5 fried mini chicken wings or drumsticks
- 1 cup chili with meat and beans

SNACKS

Choose one of the following to consume anytime of the day (but not within an hour before or after eating a meal). This is your only snack for the day, so time it wisely.

- 1 hard-boiled egg
- 10 olives
- 3.75-ounce can sardines
- 5 tortilla chips and 2 tablespoons guacamole or salsa
- Pulled-pork lettuce wrap with ⅓ cup pulled pork

EXERCISE

PM

Twenty-minute lower-intensity cardio workout or 20-minute HIIT session. Don't eat anything for at least an hour after your workout.

DAY 4
BREAKFAST

Choose one of the following:

- 1 cup oatmeal, grits, or Cream of Wheat and 2 slices of bacon

- 1 red bell pepper stuffed with cheese and 1 egg

LUNCH

Choose one of the following:

- Enchilada Bowl (page 187)
- Salmon Avocado Power Bowl (page 191)

DINNER

Choose one of the following:

- Chicken and pasta: 2 cups cooked pasta shells with sautéed chicken, sun-dried tomatoes, garlic, broccoli, and Parmesan
- Deconstructed guacamole and chicken salad: 2 cups spring mix, 3 ounces roasted chicken, tomatoes, onions, avocado, and shredded cabbage

SNACKS

Choose two of the following to consume anytime of the day (but not consecutively and not within an hour before or after eating a meal):

- 4 whole-wheat crackers and 2 servings of fat-free cheese
- 30 grapes
- 1 cup strawberries
- ⅓ cup wasabi peas
- ½ cucumber (seeded) stuffed with one thin slice of lean turkey and mustard or fat-free mayonnaise

EXERCISE

PM

Twenty-minute lower-intensity cardio workout. Don't eat anything for at least an hour after your workout (see chapter 11 for exercise examples).

DAY 5

500-CALORIE FASTING DAY

You must consume six to ten cups of no-calorie water today. This is critical. Try squeezing a little fresh lemon juice into your water to help suppress your appetite longer. You will eat only two meals and a snack, so make sure you space them properly as they need to stretch the entire day. Your calorie intake will be very low today, so adjust your physical activity accordingly. The goal is to train your body to mobilize your fat stores to be used for energy.

MEAL 1

Choose one of the following:

- 1 scrambled egg with 2 tablespoons shredded cheese
- Smoothie or protein shake (200 calories or less)
- 1 pancake, made with whole-wheat or almond flour and almond milk, and 1 slice of bacon

MEAL 2

Choose one of the following:

- 4-ounce turkey burger (no bun)
- Bacon-wrapped asparagus: 2 slices of bacon and 2 asparagus spears
- 4 pieces sushi of your choice (avocado rolls, cucumber and avocado rolls, shrimp tempura rolls, spicy tuna rolls, or California rolls)

SNACKS

Choose one of the following to consume anytime of the day (but not within an hour before or after eating a meal). This is your only snack for the day, so time it wisely.

- Crab-cake lettuce wrap: combine 6 ounces crabmeat, 2 tablespoons Greek yogurt, ¼ cup diced tomato, ⅛ cup chopped celery, salt, and pepper to taste (makes two: eat one and save the second for a snack another day)
- 10 organic seaweed snacks
- 2 Medjool dates
- ¼ avocado mashed and spread on 5 whole-wheat crackers
- Turkey lettuce wrap, with 6 ounces turkey and 2 lettuce leaves (makes two: eat one and save the second for a snack another day)

EXERCISE

AM

Twenty-minute fasted workout and lower-intensity cardio exercise (see chapter 11 for exercise examples). Don't eat anything before your workout and for at least two hours after.

DAY 6
BREAKFAST

Choose one of the following:

- 2-egg omelet with diced vegetables and 1 ounce cheese
- Avocado toast on 1 slice of whole-wheat bread

LUNCH

Choose one of the following:

- Bacon and avocado Caesar salad (add 1 slice of bacon and avocado to a regular Caesar salad)
- Garlic shrimp Caesar salad (add 3 to 5 garlic shrimp to a regular Caesar salad)

DINNER

Choose one of the following:

- 6-ounce salmon fillet sautéed with cremini mushrooms and simmered in tomato cream sauce over pasta of your choice
- Spinach ravioli: 3 ravioli (no larger than 3 inches by 2 inches) stuffed with spinach and cheese, with marinara sauce

SNACKS

Choose two of the following to consume anytime of the day (but not consecutively and not within an hour before or after eating a meal):

- 2 tablespoons sunflower seeds
- 17 pecans

- ½ cup low-fat cottage cheese mixed with 1 tablespoon natural peanut butter
- 4.5-ounce chocolate fudge sugar-free pudding with 5 sliced strawberries and a squirt of whipped cream (approximately 1 tablespoon)
- Strawberry salad: 1 cup raw spinach with ½ cup sliced strawberries and 1 tablespoon balsamic vinegar

EXERCISE

Rest day. If you still want to exercise, do a low-intensity cardio workout for 15 to 20 minutes. This will be a bonus workout, and it will help you achieve your goals faster (see chapter 11 for exercise examples).

DAY 7

BREAKFAST

Choose one of the following:

- 3 link sausages (3 to 4 inches long) and 1 cup pan-roasted vegetables
- 2 fried eggs with a slice of bacon and a side of greens

LUNCH

Choose one of the following:

- ½ cup tuna salad in a sandwich or without bread and with a cup of soup (no potato or cream)
- 5-ounce bacon cheeseburger (no bun) and a small green garden salad

DINNER

Choose one of the following:

- 6-ounce steak with a serving of creamy spinach
- 6-ounce grilled or pan-fried fish with asparagus

SNACKS

Choose two of the following to consume anytime of the day (but not consecutively and not within an hour before or after eating a meal):

- 2 ounces smoked salmon
- 6 oysters
- 5 tortilla chips and ⅓ cup guacamole
- 1 thin brown rice cake spread with 1 tablespoon peanut butter
- 2 small peaches

EXERCISE

Rest day. If you still want to exercise, do a low-intensity cardio workout for 15 to 20 minutes. This will be a bonus workout, and it will help you achieve your goals faster (see chapter 11 for exercise examples).

5

WEEK 3
CONVERSION

After two weeks of this new style of eating and exercising, you are on the threshold of a full conversion. This third week is critical: your body has been working hard to make adaptations and adjustments, and now it's ready to fully convert to the pathway of improved and sustainable metabolic flexibility and weight loss. Now that you've had a chance to sample the 5:2 method of fasting, we are going to return to the time-restricted feeding method that you followed in week 1. Your body needs to be continuously challenged to burn carbs when they're available as a fuel source and to burn fats when carbs have been depleted and are no longer available. Now that your body is familiar with the concept of fasting, we will turn it up a notch this week and make slight adjustments to your eating and fasting windows that will make your body even more efficient at burning whatever fuel is available at any given time.

GUIDELINES

Here are your guidelines for this week. The most important part of making this week a success is following the TRF method of intermittent fasting.

- **Eating Schedule.** You will have eight hours to consume all of your food and beverages with calories (eating window). The next 16 hours are going to be your fasting window. During your fast you can have as many no-calorie beverages as you like. If you want to drink beverages like coffee or tea during this period, make sure the total amount of calories you consume is no more than 50 calories. The timing of your windows is completely up to you and your schedule, but here's a sample of what a 16:8 day might look like.

FEEDING WINDOW	FASTING WINDOW
12:00 PM–8:00 PM	8:00 PM–12:00 PM

- **Water.** You must consume one cup of water before each meal. You can drink more water during and after the meal, but one cup must be consumed before your first bite.

- **Fruits and Vegetables.** They can be frozen or fresh. You can have canned fruits and vegetables, but that is the last option, as they tend to be packed with lots of salt and other preservatives. If possible, eat only vegetables and fruits with no added ingredients. If eating canned, make sure it is low-sodium (140 milligrams or less per serving).

- **Alcohol.** You're allowed to drink alcohol this week, but remember, you're trying to lose weight and improve your metabolic flexibility. Too much alcohol is going to make it that much more difficult to reach your goals. You are allowed to drink only low-carb alcohol. You can consume alcohol on the following days—days 1, 2, 3, 4, 5, 6, and 7. You are allowed only one drink on those days, either a "lite" beer or a mixed drink. The table here lists the allowed alcoholic beverages and mixers and their quantities.

TYPE OF ALCOHOL	SERVING SIZE ALLOWED
Gin	1.5 ounces (44 milliliters)
"Lite" beer	12 ounces (355 milliliters)
Red wine	5 ounces (148 milliliters)
Tequila	1.5 ounces (44 milliliters)
Vodka	1.5 ounces (44 milliliters)
Whiskey	1.5 ounces (44 milliliters)
White wine	5 ounces (148 milliliters)

TYPE OF MIXER	SERVING SIZE ALLOWED
Diet soda	½ cup
Seltzer	Unrestricted
Sugar-free tonic water	Unrestricted

- **Soda.** Neither regular nor diet soda is allowed. This is very important. If you're someone who drinks sodas, please try to eliminate them from your diet, but if you can't, at least cut your consumption in half. The one exception is diet soda as a mixer in your alcoholic beverage (see the alcohol guidelines table).

- **Sugar.** No table or cane sugar is allowed, but you can have sweeteners like organic stevia, organic monk fruit, pure or raw honey, or organic erythritol. (Be careful not to consume too much erythritol as it can cause diarrhea.)

- **Syrup.** You are allowed to use sugar-free or no-added-sugar syrups. If you can find organic syrup, then all the better.

- **Coffee.** You can have coffee during your fasting periods, but you can't load it up with calories. During your fasting period you can't consume more than 50 calories total, and adding cream and sugar to your coffee could take you over that mark. On your keto (low-carb) days, be mindful of what you put in your coffee, as you can't consume more than 50 grams of carbs for the entire day. Some coffee preparations have so many carbs that you could drink your entire day's allowance, and then some, in a single cup.

- **Meal Swaps.** Sometimes the plan might present you with meal options that you don't like, or that have ingredients you might not have access to. Don't panic. You are allowed to swap meals as long as you swap them in the same category (breakfast, lunch, dinner, meal 1, meal 2) and on the same type of day (carb-loading, 500 calories or less, and so on). For example, if you are on a keto day, then you can swap a meal from another keto day, but you can't swap for a meal from a carb-loading day. If you're on a 500-calorie-or-less fasting day, then you can swap with a similar day from within that week or another week, but you can't swap with a regular day.

- **Ingredient Elimination.** If there's an ingredient or food that you don't like, have an allergy to, or simply don't have access to, feel free to eliminate it and just use the rest of the ingredients and foods.

- **Snacks.** Please try to consume only the snacks that are listed in the daily meal plan or in chapter 10. If for some reason you need to eat a snack that's not listed, make sure it's no more than 150 calories.

- **Exercise.** The exercise is written specifically to complement the fasting method as well as the meal plan. Pay close attention to the instructions. You can find examples of the exercises in chapter 11.

DAY 1: CARB-LOADING
BREAKFAST

Choose one of the following:

- 2 cups oatmeal, grits, or Cream of Wheat with 1 slice of bacon
- 2 cups cereal (no sugar) with milk and 1 piece of fruit or ½ cup berries

LUNCH

Choose one of the following:

- 1 cup soup, such as bean, chicken noodle, tomato, squash, minestrone, or clam chowder, and a small green garden salad
- Turkey, chicken, or ham sandwich with lettuce, tomato, and cheese on the bread of your choice, with 1 tablespoon of your preferred condiment

THE INTERMITTENT FASTING HACKS: WATER, TEA, AND COFFEE

The benefits of intermittent fasting have been well studied and documented. There are millions of people around the world who have found success with this type of eating strategy. For many the adjustments required to be successful can be challenging, but the effort can pay heavy dividends. Although there are many tricks to making these adjustments, what you drink can be the easiest to implement. Water, tea, and coffee are great to drink while fasting, for three important reasons.

First, these beverages have few if any calories: black coffee has five or fewer calories, tea has no more than two, and water has zero calories. During a fast it's critical to not consume too many calories, as that will shift you out of ketosis and you will stop burning fat for fuel. Second, these beverages can help trigger a satiety signal (a feeling of fullness) in your brain, which will decrease your hunger and impulse to eat. One of the biggest goals of weight loss, and the path to success, is gaining the ability to eat fewer calories and be satisfied. Third, hydration is key. Our bodies are 70 percent water. Throughout the day and even at night, we are constantly losing water, whether in liquid form or through the air we exhale during breathing. We need to replace this water if our bodies are to continue performing optimally. This is especially true during fasting. When you're not consuming any calories, you can at least stay hydrated. That's why water, tea, and coffee— without added ingredients like cream and sugar—can be your best friends on fasting days.

DINNER

Choose one of the following:

- 2 cups spaghetti and three 1-inch meatballs in a marinara sauce
- 6-ounce piece of chicken with two servings of vegetables of your choice

SNACKS

Choose two of the following to consume anytime of the day (but not consecutively and not within an hour before or after eating a meal):

- Chickpea salad: ¼ cup chickpeas with 1 tablespoon sliced scallions, a squeeze of lemon juice, and ¼ cup diced tomato
- 1 ounce cheddar cheese with 4 to 5 radishes
- 25 peanuts, oil-roasted
- 3 tablespoons roasted unsalted soy nuts
- 2 scoops of sorbet

EXERCISE

AM OR PM

Twenty-minute HIIT session (see chapter 11 for exercise examples). Consume at least 20 grams of protein and 15 grams of carbs within an hour of finishing your workout.

DAY 2: CARB-LOADING
BREAKFAST

Choose one of the following:

- 2 pancakes (no larger than 6 inches wide) with a slice of turkey or pork bacon
- 8-ounce yogurt parfait and a small blueberry, corn, carrot, bran, or banana muffin

LUNCH

- Large green salad: 3 cups greens with 3 ounces sliced chicken, ham, or fish if desired and no more than 2 tablespoons dressing (optional additions: 5 olives, 8 halved cherry tomatoes, 2 tablespoons nuts or seeds of your choice, 8 thin cucumber slices, 3 tablespoons shredded cheese, and 4 halved strawberries)
- 2 slices of cheese, pepperoni, vegetable, or sausage pizza (each slice approximately 5 inches wide by 6 inches long) with a small green garden salad

DINNER

Choose one of the following:

- Steak salad: 6 ounces thinly sliced steak over a bed of 2 cups arugula, kale, or spinach; 1 plum tomato, cut into wedges; ½ red bell pepper, sliced; ⅓ cup sliced pineapple; and 1 tablespoon fresh lime juice
- 1 cup pasta, chicken, or fish, and vegetables in a lemon-wine or tomato-based sauce

SNACKS

Choose two of the following to consume anytime of the day (but not consecutively and not within an hour before or after eating a meal):

- Crunchy kale salad: 1 cup chopped kale leaves with 1 teaspoon honey and 1 tablespoon balsamic vinegar
- Cucumber sandwich: ½ English muffin with 2 tablespoons cottage cheese and 3 slices of cucumber
- 10 cooked mussels
- 3 ounces tuna, canned in water
- Dark chocolate and peanut butter (½-ounce dark chocolate square with 2 teaspoons organic peanut butter)

EXERCISE

AM

Twenty-minute fasted workout and lower-intensity cardio exercise (see chapter 11 for exercise examples). Don't eat anything before your workout and for at least two hours after.

PM

Twenty-minute lower-intensity cardio workout (see chapter 11 for exercise examples). Don't eat anything for at least an hour after.

DAY 3
BREAKFAST

Choose one of the following:

- Breakfast Burrito Bowl (page 146)
- 2 Bacon Egg Cups (page 144)

LUNCH

Choose one of the following:

- Chicken mayonnaise salad: chicken, avocado, cucumber, mayo, onions, tomato
- Cobb salad: 2 cups spring mix greens, 2 sliced hard-boiled eggs, roasted sweet potato slices, avocado slices, cucumber slices, halved cherry tomatoes, and roasted almonds

DINNER

Choose one of the following:

- Citrus shrimp bowl: 2 cups baby spinach or arugula, roasted shrimp cooked in a citrus glaze, red onions, halved cherry tomatoes, avocado slices, and ½ cup cooked brown rice
- 3 lamb chops with creamy spinach or asparagus

SNACKS

Choose two of the following to consume anytime of the day (but not consecutively and not within an hour before or after eating a meal):

- Avocado chips or crisps (store-bought, 150-calorie serving)
- 2 Burger Fat Bombs (page 208)
- Keto ice cream (store-bought, 150-calorie serving)
- Cheese puffs (keto-friendly, store-bought, 150-calorie serving)
- Bacon Guac Bomb (page 202)

EXERCISE

Rest day. If you still want to exercise, do a low-intensity cardio workout for 15 to 20 minutes. This will be a bonus workout, and it will help you achieve your goals faster (see chapter 11 for exercise examples).

DAY 4
BREAKFAST

Choose one of the following:

- Ham, Cheese, and Egg Rolls (page 147)
- 2 biscuits, made with almond flour, and 3 tablespoons sausage gravy

LUNCH

Choose one of the following:

- Poke Bowl (page 198)
- 1 cup chicken stir-fry and ½ cup brown rice

DINNER

Choose one of the following:

- 6-ounce Chilean sea bass in a miso glaze, cream sauce, and zucchini
- Garlic-butter steak with mushrooms and ½ cup cauliflower rice

SNACKS

Choose two of the following to consume anytime of the day (but not consecutively and not within an hour before or after eating a meal):

- Cucumber sushi
- Cookie Dough Fat Bombs (page 209)
- Bacon-Wrapped Asparagus Bites (page 205)
- Low-Carb Chocolate Chip Cookies (page 206)
- 1 hard-boiled egg

EXERCISE

AM

Twenty-minute fasted workout and lower-intensity cardio exercise (see chapter 11 for exercise examples). Don't eat anything before your workout and for at least two hours after.

PM

Fifteen-minute HIIT session (see chapter 11 for exercise examples). Don't eat anything for at least an hour after your workout.

DAY 5
BREAKFAST

Choose one of the following:

- Scrambled eggs in butter on a bed of lettuce topped with ¼ avocado, sliced
- Bell pepper stuffed with 3 ounces cheese and 1 egg

LUNCH

Choose one of the following:

- 5-ounce grass-fed beef burger (no bun) with sliced tomato and a small green salad (arugula, kale, or spinach)
- Egg salad: 2 hard-boiled eggs; ¼ celery rib, chopped; ½ teaspoon dill; ¼ yellow onion, chopped; ½ teaspoon yellow mustard; and 2 tablespoons mayonnaise

DINNER

Choose one of the following:

- Chicken breast with cauliflower mash and green beans
- 1 grilled or pan-fried pork chop and 1 cup cooked broccoli

SNACKS

Choose two of the following to consume anytime of the day (but not consecutively and not within an hour before or after eating a meal):

- Carrot sticks and guacamole
- Ham, Cheese, and Egg Rolls (page 147)
- Bacon Avocado Bomb (page 204)
- ¾ cup roasted Brussels sprouts sprinkled with a pinch of salt and extra-virgin olive oil
- Meat-Stuffed Pepper (page 210)

EXERCISE

AM OR PM

Twenty minutes of strength training (see chapter 11 for exercise examples). Consume at least 20 grams of protein and 15 grams of carbs within an hour of finishing your workout.

DAY 6
BREAKFAST

Choose one of the following:

- 1 Avocado Egg Boat (page 148)
- Two 6-inch pancakes, made with whole-wheat or almond flour and almond milk, with 2 slices of bacon

LUNCH

Choose one of the following:

- Salmon Avocado Power Bowl (page 191)
- Garlic shrimp Caesar salad (add 3 to 5 garlic shrimp to regular Caesar salad)

DINNER

Choose one of the following:

- 6-ounce grilled branzino (or another fish of your choice) in lemon-butter caper sauce with creamy spinach or broccoli
- 6-ounce skirt steak (or a different cut of your choice) in your choice of marinade with sautéed onions

SNACKS

Choose two of the following to consume anytime of the day (but not consecutively and not within an hour before or after eating a meal):

- Keto tortilla chips (store-bought, 100-calorie serving) and 2 tablespoons guacamole
- 8 to 10 zucchini fries
- 3 ounces cheddar cheese crisps, store-bought or homemade: place thinly sliced cheddar cheese on parchment paper and bake at 375°F until crisp
- ½ avocado stuffed with 3 ounces tuna or salmon
- Keto chocolate bar (store-bought, 150-calorie serving)

EXERCISE

AM

Twenty-minute fasted workout and lower-intensity cardio exercise (see chapter 11 for exercise examples). Don't eat anything before your workout and for at least two hours after.

DAY 7
BREAKFAST

Choose one of the following:

- 2 scrambled eggs in butter, with cheese if desired, and 2 slices of bacon
- 8-ounce full-fat yogurt topped with 2 tablespoons keto granola (store-bought or homemade)

LUNCH

Choose one of the following:

- Chicken Burrito Bowl (page 196)
- Grass-fed beef burger (no bun) with guacamole, tomato, and a kale salad

DINNER

Choose one of the following:

- 1 large lobster tail with butter sauce
- 6-ounce Cajun-spiced chicken breast with Brussels sprouts

SNACKS

Choose two of the following to consume anytime of the day (but not consecutively and not within an hour before or after eating a meal):

- Beef biltong (store-bought, 150-calorie serving)
- 0.4-ounce bar aged cheddar (store-bought)
- Ham, Cheese, and Egg Rolls (page 147)
- Keto brownies (store-bought, 150-calorie serving)
- BLT lettuce wrap: 2 slices of bacon, 2 slices of tomato, and 1 tablespoon shredded cheese wrapped in a large romaine lettuce leaf

EXERCISE

Rest day. If you still want to exercise, do a low-intensity cardio workout for 15 to 20 minutes. This will be a bonus workout, and it will help you achieve your goals faster (see chapter 11 for exercise examples).

6

WEEK 4
RHYTHM

You have now completed three weeks on the plan. The first thing you should do is congratulate yourself, as this is worthy of celebration. You also should be noticing real changes, whether it's the way you look, how your clothes fit, your energy levels, or your stamina. You are now in a rhythm, and it's one that you'll want to maintain so it will bring you even more results and carry you closer to your goals.

This week you will continue with the time-restricted feeding schedule of last week. Nothing will change, except that you will have a few different dietary choices. The aim of this close similarity of the fourth week to the previous week is to keep you in a rhythm. Achieving this groove is extremely beneficial: as elements of the **Met Flex Diet** plan become more familiar, they should be getting easier too. Some things you did last week that required real thought will come to you now as almost a reflex. Your body will be more open to the challenges of your workout routine because it has "been there, done that."

Your mindset this week is critical. You are crossing the midpoint as you begin the other half of your six-week journey. Sharpen your focus. Strengthen your belief. Execute with confidence, determination, and the vigor that will expand your results and carry you closer to your goals.

GUIDELINES

Here are your guidelines for this week. The TRF method of intermittent fasting you'll be following is the most important part of making this week a success.

- **Eating Schedule.** Each day you will have an eating window of eight hours in which to consume all of your food and beverages with calories. The next 16 hours will be your fasting window. During your fast you can have as many no-calorie beverages as you like; if you want to drink beverages like coffee or tea during this period, make you drink no more than a total of 50 calories. The timing of your windows is completely up to you and your schedule, but here's a sample of what a 16:8 day might look like.

FEEDING WINDOW	FASTING WINDOW
12:00 PM–8:00 PM	8:00 PM–12:00 PM

- **Water.** You must consume one cup of water before each meal. You can drink more water during and after the meal, but one cup must be consumed before your first bite.

- **Fruits and Vegetables.** They can be frozen or fresh. You can have canned, but that is the last option, as they tend to be packed with lots of salt and other preservatives. If possible, eat only vegetables and fruits with no added ingredients. If eating canned, make sure they are low-sodium (140 milligrams or less per serving).

- **Alcohol.** You're allowed to drink alcohol this week, but remember, you're trying to lose weight and improve your metabolic flexibility. Too much alcohol is going to make it that much more difficult to reach your goals. You are allowed to drink only low-carb alcohol. You can consume alcohol on the following days—days 1, 2, 3, 4, 5, 6, and 7. You are allowed only one drink on those days, either a "lite" beer or a mixed drink. The table here lists the allowed alcoholic beverages and mixers and their quantities.

TYPE OF ALCOHOL	SERVING SIZE ALLOWED
Gin	1.5 ounces (44 milliliters)
"Lite" beer	12 ounces (355 milliliters)
Red wine	5 ounces (148 milliliters)
Tequila	1.5 ounces (44 milliliters)
Vodka	1.5 ounces (44 milliliters)
Whiskey	1.5 ounces (44 milliliters)
White wine	5 ounces (148 milliliters)

TYPE OF MIXER	SERVING SIZE ALLOWED
Diet soda	½ cup
Seltzer	Unrestricted
Sugar-free tonic water	Unrestricted

- **Soda.** Neither regular nor diet soda is allowed. This is very important. If you're someone who drinks sodas, please try to eliminate them from your diet, but if you can't, at least cut your consumption in half. The one exception is diet soda as a mixer in your alcoholic beverage (see the alcohol guidelines table).

- **Sugar.** No table or cane sugar is allowed, but you can have sweeteners like organic stevia, organic monk fruit, pure or raw honey, or organic erythritol. (Be careful not to consume too much erythritol as it can cause diarrhea.)

- **Syrup.** You are allowed to use sugar-free or no-added-sugar syrups. If you can find organic syrup, then all the better.

- **Coffee.** You can have coffee during your fasting periods, but you can't load it up with calories. During your fasting period you can't consume more than 50 calories total, and adding cream and sugar to your coffee could take you over that mark. On your keto (low-carb) days, be mindful of what you put in your coffee, as you can't consume more than 50 grams of carbs for the entire day. Some coffee preparations have so many carbs that you could drink your entire day's allowance, and then some, in a single cup.

- **Meal Swaps.** Sometimes the plan might present you with meal options that you don't like, or that have ingredients you might not have access to. Don't panic. You are allowed to swap meals as long as you swap them in the same category (breakfast, lunch, dinner, meal 1, meal 2) and on the same type of day (carb-loading, 500 calories or less, and so on). For example, if you are on a keto day, then you can swap a meal from another keto day, but you can't swap for a meal from a carb-loading day. If you're on a 500-calorie-or-less fasting day, then you can swap with a similar day from that week or another week, but you can't swap for a meal from a regular day.

- **Ingredient Elimination.** If there's an ingredient or food that you don't like, have an allergy to, or simply don't have access to, feel free to eliminate it and just use the rest of the ingredients and foods.

- **Snacks.** Please try to consume only the snacks that are listed in the daily meal plan or in chapter 10. If for some reason you need to eat a snack that's not listed, make sure it's no more than 150 calories.

- **Exercise.** The exercise is written specifically to complement the fasting method as well as the meal plan. Pay close attention to the instructions. You can find examples of the exercises in chapter 11.

DAY 1: CARB-LOADING
BREAKFAST

Choose one of the following:

- 2 pancakes with 2 slices of bacon (beef or pork) and ½ cup fruit
- 2 scrambled eggs with cheese and diced vegetables

LUNCH

Choose one of the following:

- 2 slices of pizza (each slice approximately 5 inches wide by 6 inches long) and a small green garden salad

EAT BEFORE YOU EAT

Regardless of the eating or diet strategy you decide to employ to lose weight, you must be mindful of the simple physiologic fact that you gain weight when you consume more calories than you burn. Other factors, such as exercise and the timing of meals, certainly play a role in weight-loss success, but saving on calories wherever possible definitely works to your advantage.

One great diet hack to prevent yourself from overeating at meals is to "eat before you eat"—literally. One interesting study out of Pennsylvania State University looked at the impact of eating soup before a meal on the number of calories the participants consumed during the subsequent meal.[1] Before eating the meal, one group in the study was given 12 minutes to consume a bowl of soup. The other group wasn't given anything to eat before the meal; instead, they were given a magazine and instructed to read and sit quietly for 12 minutes. Once this period was over, the subjects had three minutes to rate their hunger and satiety (feelings of fullness), then all were given permission to eat as much or as little of the meal and the beverages as they liked. Not surprisingly, the researchers found that the group that ate soup first not only rated their hunger as lower before the meal but also consumed less food during the meal. Store this hack in your tool kit and don't be afraid to use it.

- 1½ cups soup, such as tomato, onion, mushroom, chicken noodle, bean, or minestrone

DINNER

Choose one of the following:

- Chicken or turkey potpie
- Lasagna (meat or meatless, 2 inches by 4 inches by 3 inches) with a small green garden salad

SNACKS

Choose two of the following to consume anytime of the day (but not consecutively and not within an hour before or after eating a meal):

- 3 pineapple rings in natural juices
- 2 cups watermelon chunks
- 4 to 5 celery sticks with 1 ounce cream cheese
- 1 cup broccoli florets with 2 tablespoons hummus
- 9 to 12 chocolate-covered almonds

EXERCISE

AM OR PM

Twenty-minute strength training or 20-minute HIIT session (see chapter 11 for exercise examples). Consume at least 20 grams of protein and 15 grams of carbs within an hour of finishing your workout.

DAY 2: CARB-LOADING
BREAKFAST

Choose one of the following:

- One 6- to 7-inch waffle with 2 slices of bacon and ½ cup berries
- 2-egg omelet with diced vegetables and 1 ounce cheese

LUNCH

Choose one of the following:

- Grilled cheese sandwich with french fries
- Large salad with 3 cups greens of your choice and 2 to 3 tablespoons dressing of your choice (optional additions: mushrooms, beets, cucumbers, rice, sunflower seeds, and basil)

DINNER

Choose one of the following:

- Large pork chop (pan-fried or grilled) with honey-glazed carrots
- 2 cups pasta, with vegetables and protein of your choice (chicken, shrimp, or seafood)

SNACKS

Choose two of the following to consume anytime of the day (but not consecutively and not within an hour before or after eating a meal):

- ½ cup roasted pumpkin seeds (in shells)
- ½ cup shelled pistachios

- ½ cup no-salt-added cottage cheese and 1 tablespoon almond butter
- 9 to 10 black olives
- ½ cup Raisin Bran (no milk)

EXERCISE

AM

Twenty-minute fasted workout and lower-intensity cardio exercise (see chapter 11 for exercise examples). Don't eat anything before your workout and for at least two hours after.

PM

Twenty-minute lower-intensity cardio workout (see chapter 11 for exercise examples). Don't eat anything for at least an hour after your workout.

DAY 3
BREAKFAST

Choose one of the following:

- 8-ounce full-fat yogurt with blueberries or strawberries topped with keto granola
- 2-egg mushroom omelet with 1 slice of bacon

LUNCH

Choose one of the following:

- Chicken Burrito Bowl (page 196)
- Steak bowl: combine 6 ounces sliced steak in a bowl with diced avocado, salsa, cauliflower rice, cherry tomatoes, and shredded cheese

DINNER

Choose one of the following:

- 3 to 4 pan-fried 2-inch crab cakes with honey mustard dipping sauce and sautéed mushrooms
- Caesar salad with 6 ounces diced skinless chicken breast, 1 slice of bacon diced, 2 cups romaine lettuce, and 2 tablespoons Caesar salad dressing or another dressing of your choice

SNACKS

Choose two of the following to consume anytime of the day (but not consecutively and not within an hour before or after eating a meal):

- 1-ounce bag of kale chips (store-bought)
- Almond butter keto cups (store-bought, 150-calorie serving)
- Cookie Dough Fat Bombs (page 209)
- 1½ cups popcorn
- Avocado Fries (page 207)

EXERCISE

Rest day. If you still want to exercise, do a low-intensity cardio workout for 15 to 20 minutes. This will be a bonus workout, and it will help you achieve your goals faster (see chapter 11 for exercise examples).

DAY 4
BREAKFAST

Choose one of the following:

- Red bell pepper stuffed with 1 scrambled egg and cheese
- 12-ounce smoothie (see chapter 9 for recipes)

LUNCH

Choose one of the following:

- Buddha Power Bowl (page 189)
- Taco salad: scoop 4 ounces cooked ground beef seasoned with 1 tablespoon taco seasoning over a bed of 2 cups greens, ⅓ cup shredded cheese, ¼ avocado, ¼ cup diced red bell pepper, and 3 tablespoons sour cream

DINNER

Choose one of the following:

- ¼ slab baby back ribs with grilled asparagus in a teriyaki or soy sauce
- Steak Tip Cacciatore with Cauliflower Rice (page 185)

SNACKS

Choose two of the following to consume anytime of the day (but not consecutively and not within an hour before or after eating a meal):

- Bacon Avocado Bomb (page 204)
- Keto tortilla chips (store-bought, 100-calorie serving) and 2 tablespoons guacamole
- 1-ounce bag of kale chips (store-bought)

- ¼ cup cinnamon toasted pumpkin seeds: in a small bowl, combine 1 ounce pumpkin seeds, 1 tablespoon extra-virgin olive oil, and ½ teaspoon cinnamon; spread on a baking sheet and bake at 325°F for 35 minutes

EXERCISE

AM

Twenty-minute fasted workout and lower-intensity cardio exercise (see chapter 11 for exercise examples). Don't eat anything before your workout and for at least two hours after.

PM

Fifteen-minute lower-intensity cardio workout. Don't eat anything for at least an hour after your workout (see chapter 11 for exercise examples).

DAY 5
BREAKFAST

Choose one of the following:

- 3 sausage links (3 to 4 inches long) and 1 cup pan-roasted vegetables
- Keto-friendly blueberry muffin (less than 6 grams of carbs) and 6 ounces full-fat yogurt

LUNCH

Choose one of the following:

- Meatball Bowl (page 193)
- Tuna salad with tomato, avocado, and macadamia nuts

DINNER

Choose one of the following:

- 6-ounce steak (cut of your choice) with creamy spinach, grilled asparagus, or broccoli
- 6-ounce fish (grilled or pan-fried) with creamy spinach, grilled asparagus, or broccoli

SNACKS

Choose two of the following to consume anytime of the day (but not consecutively and not within an hour before or after eating a meal):

- 3 blue cheese–stuffed apricots: cut apricots in half and remove pits; in a small bowl, mix ⅓ cup blue cheese crumbles, ⅛ teaspoon salt, and 2 teaspoons extra-virgin olive oil; stuff apricot halves with blue cheese mix, then place on parchment paper on a baking sheet and bake at 375°F for 2 to 3 minutes
- No-sugar-added jerky (store-bought, 150-calorie serving)
- Keto peanut butter cookies (store-bought, 150-calorie serving)
- 10 organic seaweed snacks

EXERCISE

AM OR PM

Twenty-minute HIIT session (see chapter 11 for exercise examples). Consume at least 20 grams of protein and 15 grams of carbs within an hour of finishing your workout.

DAY 6
BREAKFAST

Choose one of the following:

- Avocado breakfast bowl: ½ avocado, 1 cup chopped lettuce, 1 small beet peeled and grated, 1 small carrot peeled and grated, 1 cup chopped cucumber, freshly squeezed juice from half a lemon, sea salt and black pepper to taste, 1 tablespoon tahini
- 12-ounce smoothie (see chapter 9 for recipes)

LUNCH

Choose one of the following:

- Deconstructed Egg Roll (page 190)
- 5-ounce beef burger (no bun) with tomato, cheese, and lettuce

DINNER

Choose one of the following:

- Stir-fried chicken breast with cauliflower mash and green beans
- Stir-fried chicken, broccoli, mushrooms, and peppers (optional: satay or peanut sauce)

SNACKS

Choose two of the following to consume anytime of the day (but not consecutively and not within an hour before or after eating a meal):

- Keto protein bar (store-bought, 150-calorie serving)
- Keto tortilla chips (store-bought, 150-calorie serving)
- Salmon cucumber bites: spread whipped cream cheese on 5 cucumber slices, then top with a small piece of smoked salmon, pepper, salt, and chopped chives
- 1 hard-boiled egg
- ¾ cup roasted Brussels sprouts

EXERCISE

AM

Twenty-minute fasted workout and lower-intensity cardio exercise (see chapter 11 for exercise examples). Don't eat anything before your workout and for at least two hours after.

DAY 7
BREAKFAST

Choose one of the following:

- Crustless Bacon, Zucchini, and Pepper Jack Quiche (page 140)
- Ham, egg, and cheese without bread

LUNCH

Choose one of the following:

- Poke Bowl (page 198)

- 5-ounce chicken or turkey burger (no bun) with lettuce, tomato, and cheese and ½ cup soup (no cream, potato, or bean)

DINNER

Choose one of the following:

- Creamy Garlic Parmesan Zucchini Noodles with Shrimp (page 174)
- 3 small lamb chops with roasted Brussels sprouts or green beans

SNACKS

Choose two of the following to consume anytime of the day (but not consecutively and not within an hour before or after eating a meal):

- 10 cheese crisps (store-bought or homemade, 150-calorie serving)
- Keto brownies (store-bought, 150-calorie serving)
- 2 cups keto popcorn
- Cheddar-flavored almond flour crackers (store-bought, 150-calorie serving)
- Keto peanut butter cookies (store-bought, 150-calorie serving]

EXERCISE

Rest day. If you still want to exercise, do a low-intensity cardio workout for 15 to 20 minutes. This will be a bonus workout, and it will help you achieve your goals faster (see chapter 11 for exercise examples).

7

WEEK 5
STRIDE

The finish line is near. Week 5 is a great opportunity to look back over the last four weeks and reflect on all of your struggles and successes, both of which are equally important, as they teach you different lessons that can be helpful on the rest of your journey. You are no longer a novice, and if you ever doubted yourself, the fact that you are reading this sentence means you have made it through and now should be in full stride.

This week will be similar to week 2 in that you will be following the 5:2 method. You've done it before, so there shouldn't be any surprises this week. The next 14 days are critical to achieving your best results. Now is not the time to pause or go backward. Harness the momentum you've built thus far, as it will push you forward and closer to the finish line.

GUIDELINES

Here are your guidelines for this week. You are going to be following the 5:2 method of intermittent fasting, so be prepared for those fasting days. The low-calorie days are spaced apart so that you will not be struggling through consecutive fasting days.

- **Eating Schedule.** You will have five days of relatively normal eating and two days of low-calorie eating (fasting). Don't switch the days in the plan, as they are in a particular order for good reason. On your fasting days, I strongly encourage you not to eat on the run, but rather to take the time to sit down in a relaxed setting and to eat and savor your food.

- **Water.** You must consume one cup of water before each meal. You can have more water during and after the meal, but one cup must be consumed before your first bite.

- **Fruits and Vegetables.** They can be frozen or fresh. You can have canned, but that is the last option, as they tend to be packed with lots of salt and other preservatives. If possible, eat vegetables and fruits with no added ingredients. If eating canned, make sure they are low-sodium (140 milligrams or less per serving).

- **Alcohol.** You're allowed to drink alcohol this week, but remember, you're trying to lose weight and improve your metabolic flexibility. Too much alcohol is going to make it that much more difficult to reach your goals. You are allowed to drink only low-carb alcohol. You can consume alcohol on the following days—days 1, 2, 4, 6, and 7. You are allowed only one drink on those days, either a "lite" beer or a mixed drink. The table here lists the allowed alcoholic beverages and mixers and their quantities.

TYPE OF ALCOHOL	SERVING SIZE ALLOWED
Gin	1.5 ounces (44 milliliters)
"Lite" beer	12 ounces (355 milliliters)
Red wine	5 ounces (148 milliliters)
Tequila	1.5 ounces (44 milliliters)
Vodka	1.5 ounces (44 milliliters)
Whiskey	1.5 ounces (44 milliliters)
White wine	5 ounces (148 milliliters)

TYPE OF MIXER	SERVING SIZE ALLOWED
Diet soda	½ cup
Seltzer	Unrestricted
Sugar-free tonic water	Unrestricted

- **Soda.** Neither regular nor diet soda is allowed. This is very important. If you're someone who drinks sodas, please try to eliminate them from your diet, but if you can't, at least cut your consumption in half. The one exception is diet soda as a mixer in your alcoholic beverage (see the alcohol guidelines table).

- **Sugar.** No table or cane sugar is allowed, but you can have sweeteners like organic stevia, organic monk fruit, pure or raw honey, or organic erythritol. (Be careful not to consume too much erythritol as it can cause diarrhea.)

- **Syrup.** You are allowed to use sugar-free or no-added-sugar syrups. If you can find organic syrup, then all the better.

- **Coffee.** You can have coffee during your fasting periods, but you can't load it up with calories. During your fasting period you can't consume more than 50 calories total, so adding cream and sugar to your coffee could take you over that mark. On your keto (low-carb) days, be mindful of what you put into your coffee, as you can't consume more than 50 grams of carbs for the entire day. Some coffee preparations have so many carbs that you could drink your entire day's allowance, and then some, in a single cup.

- **Meal Swaps.** Sometimes the plan might present you with meal options that you don't like, or that have ingredients you might not have access to. Don't panic. You are allowed to swap meals as long as you swap them in the same category (breakfast, lunch, dinner, meal 1, meal 2) and on the same type of day (carb-loading, 500 calories or less, and so on). For example, if you are on a keto day, then you can swap a meal from another keto day, but you can't swap for a meal from a carb-loading day. If you're on a 500-calorie-or-less fasting day, then you can swap with a similar day from within that week or another week, but you can't swap with a regular day.

- **Ingredient Elimination.** If there's an ingredient or food that you don't like, have an allergy to, or simply don't have access to, feel free to eliminate it and just use the rest of the ingredients and foods.

- **Snacks.** Please try to consume only the snacks listed in the daily meal plan or in chapter 10. If for some reason you need to eat a snack that's not listed, please make sure it's no more than 150 calories. On the two fasting days, you will be allowed to have one snack from those that are listed, so choose wisely, as it will be critical in helping you stretch your calories throughout the day as best as possible.

- **Exercise.** The exercise is written specifically to complement the fasting method as well as the meal plan. Pay close attention to the instructions. You can find examples of the exercises in chapter 11.

DAY 1: CARB-LOADING
BREAKFAST

Choose one of the following:

- 1 cup oatmeal, grits, or Cream of Wheat and 1 piece of fruit
- Breakfast smoothie or protein shake (300 calories or less)

LUNCH

Choose one of the following:

- Spaghetti and meatballs (2 cups cooked pasta and 2 meatballs) in a tomato-based sauce
- Large salad with 3 cups greens of your choice and 2 to 3 tablespoons dressing of your choice (optional additions: mushrooms, beets, cucumbers, rice, sunflower seeds, and basil)

LESS STRESS,
LESS MESS

Stress is more than just an abstract concept. It's a specific phenomenon with specific implications for your physical and mental well-being. Scientific literature is rife with studies that have shown the impact of stress on weight gain and weight loss. Stress can have a physiologic impact on almost every area of the body, affecting various functions and even cellular processes. Even if you follow a diet and exercise plan, stress-related changes can cause you to experience several factors that lead to weight gain, such as cravings for unhealthy, high-calorie foods, decreased motivation to be physically active, increased appetite, and poor sleep. Some of the strategies you can try to reduce your stress are meditating, listening to music, reading a book, practicing mindfulness, creating better time management practices, engaging in hobbies, and practicing breathing and relaxation techniques. Getting more sleep, spending more time on things that give you pleasure, and avoiding excessive consumption of caffeine can help relieve the anxiety of stress and give your body a chance to recalibrate and settle.

DINNER

Choose one of the following:

- Vegetarian plate: 4 servings of cooked or raw vegetables (1 serving is about ½ cup cooked vegetables) and 1 cup rice
- Grilled chicken breast with mashed potatoes and peas (or another veggie of your choice)

SNACKS

Choose two of the following to consume anytime of the day (but not consecutively and not within an hour before or after eating a meal):

- 5 frozen yogurt–dipped strawberries (dip strawberries in yogurt, then freeze)
- 1 medium grapefruit sprinkled with ½ teaspoon sugar and broiled if desired
- ⅔ cup sugar snap peas and 3 tablespoons hummus
- Small (4.5-ounce) chocolate pudding
- 1 cup grape tomatoes and 6 whole-wheat crackers

EXERCISE

AM

Twenty-minute fasted workout and lower-intensity cardio exercise (see chapter 11 for exercise examples). Don't eat anything for at least two hours after the workout.

DAY 2: CARB-LOADING
BREAKFAST

Choose one of the following:

- 1½ cups cold cereal (no sugar) with milk and a piece of fruit
- One 8-inch waffle or two 4-inch waffles with 2 slices of bacon (pork or turkey), two 3-inch link sausages, or one 3-inch-wide sausage patty (optional additions: butter and syrup)

LUNCH

Choose one of the following:

- 5-ounce cheeseburger (with bun) with french fries
- 2 slices of cheese, pepperoni, or veggie pizza (each slice approximately 5 inches wide by 6 inches long)

DINNER

Choose one of the following:

- Masala-Dusted Chicken Thighs with Garlicky Brown Butter Spinach (page 159)
- 2 cups whole-wheat pasta, 3 ounces diced chicken, and tomatoes and broccoli

SNACKS

Choose two of the following to consume anytime of the day (but not consecutively and not within an hour before or after eating a meal):

- 7 saltines
- Spicy black beans: ¼ cup black beans with 1 tablespoon salsa and 1 tablespoon fat-free Greek yogurt
- 4 ounces chicken breast wrapped in lettuce and topped with dill mustard
- Turkey wrap: 2 slices of deli turkey breast, sliced tomatoes and cucumbers, and lettuce wrapped in whole-grain flatbread
- 1½ cups puffed rice

EXERCISE

AM

Twenty-minute fasted workout, lower-intensity cardio exercises, and 15 minutes of strength training (see chapter 11 for exercise examples). Don't eat anything before your workout or for at least two hours after.

DAY 3

500-CALORIE FASTING DAY

You must consume six to ten cups of no-calorie water today. This is critical. Try squeezing a little fresh lemon juice into the water to help suppress your appetite longer. You will have only two meals and a snack, so make sure you space them properly, as they need to stretch the entire day. Your calorie intake will be very low today, so adjust your physical activity accordingly. The goal is to train your body to mobilize your fat stores to be used for energy.

MEAL 1

Choose one of the following:

- 1 Keto Pancake (page 142) and 1 slice of bacon
- 1 scrambled egg with cheese and 1 slice of bacon
- 8-ounce full-fat yogurt with strawberries and 1 tablespoon granola

MEAL 2

Choose one of the following:

- Low-Carb Burger Bowl (page 195)
- 1 cup soup, such as chicken noodle, minestrone, tomato, broccoli cheddar, creamy mushroom, creamy asparagus, roasted cauliflower, or French onion (totaling no more than 12 grams of carbs), and a small green garden salad
- 1 cup chili

SNACK

Choose one of the following to consume anytime of the day (but not within an hour before or after eating a meal). This is your only snack for the day, so time it wisely.

- 2 Burger Fat Bombs (page 208)
- Keto ice cream (store-bought, 150-calorie serving, less than 3 grams of carbs per serving)
- 3 ounces cheddar cheese crisps (store-bought or homemade)
- ½ avocado stuffed with 3 ounces tuna or salmon
- Two 0.4-ounce bars aged cheddar (store-bought)

EXERCISE

PM

Twenty-minute lower-intensity cardio workout. Don't eat anything for at least an hour after your workout (see chapter 11 for exercise examples).

DAY 4
BREAKFAST

Choose one of the following:

- 1 slice of egg frittata
- Breakfast Burrito Bowl (page 146)

LUNCH

Choose one of the following:

- Philly Cheese Steak Bowl (page 199)
- 8 to 10 fried mini chicken wings or drumsticks

DINNER

Choose one of the following:

- Almond and Chicharrones–Crusted Pork Tenderloin with Chipotle Cauliflower Smash (page 151)
- 6 ounces grilled or pan-fried fish, 1 cup cooked green beans, and ½ cup cooked cauliflower rice

SNACKS

Choose two of the following to consume anytime of the day (but not consecutively and not within an hour before or after eating a meal):

- 25 peanuts, oil-roasted
- 21 raw almonds
- BLT lettuce wrap: 2 slices of bacon, 2 slices of tomato, and 1 tablespoon shredded cheese wrapped in a large romaine lettuce leaf
- 1 dill pickle wrapped in turkey or ham
- Avocado chips (store-bought, 150-calorie serving)

EXERCISE

AM OR PM

Twenty-minute strength training or 20-minute HIIT workout (see chapter 11 for exercise examples). Consume at least 20 grams of protein and 15 grams of carbs within an hour of finishing your workout.

DAY 5

500-CALORIE FASTING DAY

You must consume six to ten cups of no-calorie water today. This is critical. Try squeezing a little fresh lemon juice into the water to help suppress your appetite longer. You will have only two meals and a snack, so make sure you space them properly as they need to stretch the entire day. Your calorie intake will be very low today, so adjust your physical activity accordingly. The goal is to train your body to mobilize your fat stores to be used for energy.

MEAL 1

Choose one of the following:

- 1 scrambled egg with cheese
- One 6-inch Keto Pancake (page 142) and 1 slice of bacon
- Grilled or baked chicken breast and green beans or broccoli

MEAL 2

Choose one of the following:

- 1 cup soup, such as chicken noodle, minestrone, tomato, broccoli cheddar, creamy mushroom, creamy asparagus, roasted cauliflower, or French onion (totaling no more than 12 grams of carbs)
- 4-ounce turkey burger (no bun)
- 5 fried mini chicken wings or drumsticks

SNACK

Choose two of the following to consume anytime of the day (but not consecutively and not within an hour before or after eating a meal):

- 17 pecans
- Cucumber sushi
- Bacon-Wrapped Asparagus Bites (page 205)

- Avocado Fries (page 207)
- Beef biltong (store-bought, 150-calorie serving)

EXERCISE

AM

Twenty minutes of strength training (see chapter 11 for exercise examples). Consume at least 20 grams of protein and 15 grams of carbs within an hour of finishing your workout.

PM

Twenty-minute lower-intensity cardio workout. Don't eat anything for at least an hour after your workout (see chapter 11 for exercise examples).

DAY 6
BREAKFAST

Choose one of the following:

- 8-ounce full-fat yogurt with berries and 2 tablespoons granola
- 12-ounce smoothie (see chapter 9 for recipes)

LUNCH

Choose one of the following:

- 6 ounces pan-fried fish of your choice and 1 cup cooked Brussels sprouts
- 4 ounces beef teriyaki and 1 cup cooked cauliflower rice or roasted cauliflower

DINNER

Choose one of the following:

- Roasted Citrus-Miso Salmon and Green Beans (page 170)
- 6-ounce steak (your choice of cut) and green beans

SNACKS

Choose two of the following to consume anytime of the day (but not consecutively and not within an hour before or after eating a meal):

- 10 organic seaweed snacks
- Keto protein bar (store-bought, 150-calorie serving)
- Turkey sticks (like beef jerky, but made with turkey; store-bought, 150-calorie serving)
- Meat-Stuffed Pepper (page 210)
- Keto chocolate chip cookies (150 calories or less if store-bought)

EXERCISE

Rest day. If you still want to exercise, do a low-intensity cardio workout for 15 to 20 minutes. This will be a bonus workout, and it will help you achieve your goals faster (see chapter 11 for exercise examples).

DAY 7
BREAKFAST

Choose one of the following:

- Chive and Gruyère Frittata with Crab and Avocado (page 138)
- Mediterranean omelet made with 2 eggs, spinach, tomatoes, Kalamata olives, and blue cheese

LUNCH

Choose one of the following:

- 5-ounce bacon cheeseburger (no bun) and a small green garden salad
- 6 ounces fish (grilled or pan-fried) and a small green garden salad

DINNER

Choose one of the following:

- Crispy Roasted Cauliflower Steaks with Zucchini "Ghanoush" (page 175)
- 2 small pan-fried, thinly cut pork chops and creamy spinach

SNACKS

Choose two of the following to consume anytime of the day (but not consecutively and not within an hour before or after eating a meal):

- Cucumber sushi
- Cookie Dough Fat Bombs (page 209)
- No-sugar-added beef jerky (store-bought, 150-calorie serving)
- 2 cups keto popcorn
- Two 0.4-ounce bars aged cheddar (store-bought)

EXERCISE

Rest day. If you still want to exercise, do a low-intensity cardio workout for 15 to 20 minutes. This will be a bonus workout, and it will help you achieve your goals faster (see chapter 11 for exercise examples.

8

WEEK 6
DOWNHILL

You are now on the steepest part of your descent toward the finish line. All of the hard work you've done the last five weeks has created momentum that, combined with your determination and (hopefully) excitement, will push you across the finish line at the end of this week. Remember, however, that finishing the **Met Flex Diet** plan doesn't mean everything stops and you return to your old behaviors and decisions just because you've finished day seven of this week. One of the important purposes of this week is to piece together all of the accumulated knowledge, experience, and familiarity so that you can make permanent lifestyle changes that will make the results you've achieved long-lasting.

You will finish this last week with a method of intermittent fasting that you haven't seen yet in the program—alternate-day fasting. Get ready for three fasting days and four regular eating days. This will be challenging, but given what you've already done, you should be able to see it through to the end with vigor.

GUIDELINES

Here are your guidelines for this week. You are going to be following the alternate day method of intermittent fasting, so be mindful and prepared for those fasting days. You will have three 500-calorie days this week, and they will not be consecutive. Be mindful of when these days are approaching and make sure you are prepared, as that is vital to your success on these days.

- **Eating Schedule.** You will have four days of relatively normal eating and three days of low-calorie eating (fasting). Don't switch the days in the program, as they are in a particular order for good reason. On your fasting days, I strongly encourage you not to eat on the run, but rather to take the time to sit down in a relaxed setting and to eat and savor your food.

- **Water.** You must consume one cup of water before each meal. You can have more water during and after the meal, but one cup must be consumed before your first bite.

- **Fruits and Vegetables.** They can be frozen or fresh. You can have canned, but that is the last option as they tend to be packed with lots of salt and other preservatives. If possible, eat vegetables and fruits with no added ingredients. If eating canned, make sure it's low-sodium (140 milligrams or less per serving).

- **Alcohol.** You're allowed to drink alcohol this week, but remember, you're trying to lose weight and improve your metabolic flexibility. Too much alcohol is going to make it that much more difficult to reach your goals. You are allowed to drink only low-carb alcohol. You can consume alcohol on the following days—days 1, 3, 5, and 7. You are allowed only one drink on those days, either a "lite" beer or a mixed drink. The table here lists the allowed alcoholic beverages and mixers and their quantities.

If you want to drink alcohol, try to limit your consumption to three glasses of wine and three beers per week. You can have only one alcoholic beverage per day, and saving up to have multiple drinks at once is not allowed. On the three fasting days, you are not allowed to have alcohol, as you need to save those calories for true nourishment from your meals and snack.

TYPE OF ALCOHOL	SERVING SIZE ALLOWED
Gin	1.5 ounces (44 milliliters)
"Lite" beer	12 ounces (355 milliliters)
Red wine	5 ounces (148 milliliters)
Tequila	1.5 ounces (44 milliliters)
Vodka	1.5 ounces (44 milliliters)
Whiskey	1.5 ounces (44 milliliters)
White wine	5 ounces (148 milliliters)

TYPE OF MIXER	SERVING SIZE ALLOWED
Diet soda	½ cup
Seltzer	Unrestricted
Sugar-free tonic water	Unrestricted

- **Soda.** Neither regular nor diet soda is allowed. This is very important. If you're someone who drinks sodas, please try to eliminate them from your diet, but if you can't, at least cut your consumption in half. The one exception is diet soda as a mixer in your alcoholic beverage (see the alcohol guidelines table).

- **Sugar.** No table or cane sugar is allowed, but you can have sweeteners like organic stevia, organic monk fruit, pure or raw honey, or organic erythritol. (Be careful not to consume too much erythritol as it can cause diarrhea.)

- **Syrup.** You are allowed to use sugar-free or no-added-sugar syrups. If you can find organic syrup, then all the better.

- **Coffee.** You can have coffee during your fasting periods, but you can't load it up with calories. During your fasting period you can't consume more than 50 calories total, so adding cream and sugar to your coffee could take you over that mark. On your keto (low-carb) days, be mindful of what you put into your coffee, as you can't consume more than 50 grams of carbs for the entire day. Some coffee preparations have so many carbs that you could drink your entire day's allowance, and then some, in a single cup.

- **Meal Swaps.** Sometimes the plan might present you with meal options that you don't like, or that have ingredients you might not have access to. Don't panic. You are allowed to swap meals as long as you swap them in the same category (breakfast, lunch, dinner, meal 1, meal 2) and on the same type of day (carb-loading, 500 calories or less, and so on). For example, if you are on a keto day, you can swap a meal from another keto day, but you can't swap for a meal from a carb-loading day. If you're on a 500-calorie-or-less fasting day, then you can swap with a similar day from within that week or another week, but you can't swap with a regular day.

- **Ingredient Elimination.** If there's an ingredient or food that you don't like, have an allergy to, or simply don't have access to, feel free to eliminate it and just use the rest of the ingredients and foods.

- **Snacks.** Please try to consume only the snacks listed in the daily meal plan or in chapter 10. If for some reason you need to eat a snack that's not listed, please make sure it's no more than 150 calories. On the three fasting days, you will be allowed to have one snack from those that are listed, so choose wisely, as it will be critical in helping you stretch your calories throughout the day as best as possible.

- **Exercise.** The exercise is written specifically to complement the fasting method as well as the meal plan. Pay close attention to the instructions. You can find examples of the exercises in chapter 11.

DAY 1: CARB-LOADING
BREAKFAST

Choose one of the following:

- One 8-inch waffle with 2 slices of bacon and ½ cup berries
- 2-egg omelet with diced vegetables and 1 ounce cheese

CHANGE YOUR CLOTHES

An enormous part of weight loss and behavioral change is mental. You might have the best intentions, you might understand what needs to be done, and you might have all the necessary resources and support to make improvements. If your mind isn't in the right space, however, your chances of maximal success are greatly diminished. As you make positive changes in your lifestyle and your body begins to change as a result of that hard work, it's important that you acknowledge your progress not only in words but also in actions. So often, people lose a significant amount of weight—enough weight to make their clothes too large or ill-fitting—yet they continue to wear these old clothes and refuse to buy new ones. For some people, financial challenges might prevent them from changing their wardrobe, but many people simply can't mentally shift their view of themselves and of their future if they continue with the positive lifestyle changes they've made.

It's critical to your long-term success that you stop seeing yourself as you were 30 or 40 pounds ago. You've worked and sacrificed and struggled to shred those pounds, and you should be proud of your success and feel confident that you can keep it off. The act of buying new clothes and getting rid of the old ones is a statement not just to yourself but to others who know you. Not only do new clothes acknowledge your success, but they provide critical inspiration and motivation to continue down your new path and not return to the old habits and environment that prompted you to make a change in the first place. To make the process an even more complete experience—and get a double dose of happiness—donate your old clothes to charity.

LUNCH

Choose one of the following:

- 5-ounce cheeseburger and french fries
- Turkey, chicken, or ham sandwich (optional additions: lettuce, cheese, and tomato) and a small green garden salad

DINNER

Choose one of the following:

- 6-ounce piece of grilled or baked chicken or fish and 2 servings of vegetables of your choice
- 2 cups cooked pasta in a marinara or lemon sauce with your choice of vegetables and optional 3 ounces chicken, steak, or fish

SNACKS

Choose two of the following to consume anytime of the day (but not consecutively and not within an hour before or after eating a meal):

- 6 dried figs
- 25 frozen red seedless grapes
- 1 cup blueberries with a squirt (1 tablespoon) of whipped cream
- 5 cucumber slices topped with ⅓ cup cottage cheese and salt and pepper
- ½ cup unsweetened applesauce mixed with 10 pecan halves

EXERCISE

AM

Twenty-minute fasted workout and lower-intensity cardio exercise (see chapter 11 for exercise examples). Don't eat anything before your workout and for at least two hours after.

PM

Fifteen-minute HIIT session. Don't eat anything for at least an hour after your workout (see chapter 11 for exercise examples).

DAY 2: CARB-LOADING

500-CALORIE FASTING DAY

You must consume six to ten cups of no-calorie water today. This is critical. Try squeezing a little fresh lemon juice into the water to help suppress your appetite longer. You will have only two meals and a snack, so make sure you space them properly, as they need to stretch the entire day. Your calorie intake will be very low today, so adjust your physical activity accordingly. The goal is to train your body to mobilize your fat stores to be used for energy.

MEAL 1

Choose one of the following:

- 8-ounce yogurt parfait with blueberries or strawberries and 1 tablespoon granola
- 1 scrambled egg with cheese and 1 slice of bacon
- 1 serving of Breakfast Burrito Bowl (page 146)

MEAL 2

Choose one of the following:

- 1 cup soup, such as chicken noodle, minestrone, tomato, broccoli cheddar, creamy mushroom, creamy asparagus, roasted cauliflower, or French onion (with no more than 12 grams of carbs) and a small green garden salad

- 2-ounce beef burger (no bun) with lettuce, tomato, and cheese

- Tuna salad: 2 ounces tuna, 8 Brussels sprouts, 2 cups arugula or spinach leaves, 3 olives, 1 hard-boiled egg, and 2 tablespoons salad dressing

SNACK

Choose one of the following to consume anytime of the day (but not within an hour before or after eating a meal). This is your only snack for the day, so time it wisely.

- 4 saltine jelly sandwiches: sugar-free jelly between 2 saltine crackers (8 crackers in all)

- Peanut butter and jelly: 1 tablespoon organic peanut butter and sugar-free jelly on ½ whole-grain English muffin

- Dark chocolate and peanut butter: ½-ounce dark chocolate square with 2 teaspoons organic peanut butter

- 2 cups air-popped popcorn with 1 teaspoon butter

EXERCISE

AM OR PM

Twenty minutes of strength training or 20-minute HIIT session (see chapter 11 for exercise examples). Consume at least 20 grams of protein and 15 grams of carbs within an hour of finishing your workout.

DAY 3
BREAKFAST

Choose one of the following:

- 2 scrambled eggs in butter on a bed of lettuce topped with avocado
- Bell pepper stuffed with cheese and eggs

LUNCH

Choose one of the following:

- Mediterranean Chicken Skewers with Shaved Carrot and Walnut Salad (page 165)
- Cobb salad: 2 cups spring mix greens; 2 hard-boiled eggs, sliced; roasted sweet potato slices; avocado slices; cucumber slices; halved cherry tomatoes; and roasted almonds

DINNER

Choose one of the following:

- Pan-Seared Pork Chops with Romesco Butter and Manchego Broccoli (page 155)
- 6 ounces Chilean sea bass in a miso glaze, with cream sauce and zucchini

SNACKS

Choose two of the following to consume anytime of the day (but not consecutively and not within an hour before or after eating a meal):

- Pork rinds/cracklins (store-bought, 150-calorie serving)
- 21 raw almonds
- Smoked bacon bits (store-bought, 150-calorie serving)
- Turkey sticks (store-bought, 150-calorie serving)
- Keto granola bar (store-bought, 150-calorie serving)

EXERCISE

AM

Twenty-minute fasted workout and lower-intensity cardio exercise (see chapter 11 for exercise examples). Don't eat anything before your workout and for at least two hours after.

PM

Twenty-minute lower-intensity cardio workout. Don't eat anything for at least an hour after your workout (see chapter 11 for exercise examples).

DAY 4

500-CALORIE FASTING DAY

You must consume six to ten cups of no-calorie water today. This is critical. Try squeezing a little fresh lemon juice into the water to help suppress your appetite longer. You will have only two meals and a snack, so make sure you space them properly, as they need to stretch the entire day. Your calorie intake will be very low today, so adjust your physical activity accordingly. The goal is to train your body to mobilize your fat stores to be used for energy.

MEAL 1

Choose one of the following:

- 1½ cups soup, such as tomato, cucumber, chicken, squash, black bean, white bean, lentil, or turkey, with a small green garden salad and 1 tablespoon dressing
- 12-ounce smoothie (200 calories or less)
- 1 scrambled egg and 1 slice of bacon

MEAL 2

Choose one of the following:

- Turkey-stuffed bell pepper: cook ¼ pound ground turkey with 1 teaspoon taco seasoning mix; cut yellow or red bell pepper in half, removing the stem, seeds, and ribs; fill the halves with the cooked turkey meat, and ½ tomato, chopped, and ¼ cup chopped lettuce divided between them; top each half with 1 tablespoon shredded cheese; bake at 350°F for approximately 5 minutes or until the cheese is melted; serve warm
- 3 ounces Chili-Rubbed Flank Steak with Chipotle Butter and Charred Lime Broccoli (page 181)
- 1 cup zucchini spaghetti: make zucchini noodles from 1 whole zucchini; sauté in extra-virgin olive oil over high heat; in a small saucepan, combine

1½ teaspoons mayonnaise, 1 teaspoon garlic powder, freshly squeezed juice from half a lemon, 1 teaspoon chopped basil, and 1 teaspoon sweetener and cook for a few minutes until a sauce forms; pour sauce over zucchini pasta and serve

SNACK

Choose one of the following to consume anytime of the day (but not within an hour before or after eating a meal). This is your only snack for the day, so time it wisely.

- Cookie Dough Fat Bombs (page 209)
- Keto crackers (store-bought, in a variety of flavors, labeled "keto-friendly," 150-calorie serving)
- 25 peanuts, oil-roasted
- Ham, Cheese, and Egg Rolls (page 147)
- 10 cheese crisps (store-bought, 150-calorie serving)

EXERCISE

AM OR PM

Twenty minutes of strength training (see chapter 11 for exercise examples). Consume at least 20 grams of protein and 15 grams of carbs within an hour of finishing your workout.

DAY 5
BREAKFAST

Choose one of the following:

- Three 3- to 4-inch sausage links and 1 cup pan-roasted vegetables

- 2-egg omelet with cheese, diced vegetables, and ham or sausage

LUNCH

Choose one of the following:

- Bacon and avocado Caesar salad
- Garlic shrimp Caesar salad

DINNER

Choose one of the following:

- Curried Coconut Cod, Shrimp, and Fennel Stew (page 172)
- 3 small lamb chops with 1 cup roasted Brussels sprouts or 1 cup green beans

SNACKS

Choose two of the following to consume anytime of the day (but not consecutively and not within an hour before or after eating a meal):

- 1 dill pickle wrapped in turkey or ham
- Pepperette meat sticks (store bought, 150-calorie serving)
- Almond butter keto cups (store-bought, 150-calorie serving)
- Almond butter squeeze pack (store-bought, 150-calorie serving)
- Keto peanut butter cookies (store-bought, 150-calorie serving)

EXERCISE

AM

Twenty-minute fasted workout and lower-intensity cardio exercise (see chapter 11 for exercise examples). Don't eat anything before your workout and for at least two hours after.

PM

Twenty-minute lower-intensity cardio workout. Don't eat anything for at least an hour after your workout (see chapter 11 for exercise examples).

DAY 6

500-CALORIE FASTING DAY

You must consume six to ten cups of no-calorie water today. This is critical. Try squeezing a little fresh lemon juice into the water to help suppress your appetite longer. You will have only two meals and a snack, so make sure you space them properly, as they need to stretch the entire day. Your calorie intake will be very low today, so adjust your physical activity accordingly. The goal is to train your body to mobilize your fat stores to be used for energy.

MEAL 1

Choose one of the following:

- 1 scrambled egg with 2 tablespoons shredded cheese
- Smoothie or protein shake (200 calories or less)
- 1 pancake, made with whole-wheat or almond flour and almond milk, and 1 slice of bacon

MEAL 2

Choose one of the following:

- 4-ounce turkey burger (no bun)
- 2 asparagus spears wrapped in 2 slices of bacon
- 4 pieces of sushi (avocado rolls, cucumber and avocado rolls, shrimp tempura rolls, spicy tuna rolls, California rolls)

SNACK

Choose one of the following to consume anytime of the day (but not within an hour before or after eating a meal). This is your only snack for the day, so time it wisely.

- Bacon Avocado Bomb (page 204)
- Meat-Stuffed Pepper (page 210)
- Keto tortilla chips (100-calorie serving) and 2 tablespoons guacamole
- 8 to 10 zucchini fries

EXERCISE

Rest day. If you still want to exercise, do a low-intensity cardio workout for 15 to 20 minutes. This will be a bonus workout, and it will help you achieve your goals faster (see chapter 11 for exercise examples).

DAY 7
BREAKFAST

Choose one of the following:

- Keto-friendly blueberry muffin and 6 ounces full-fat yogurt
- 2 scrambled eggs with cheese and diced vegetables

LUNCH

Choose one of the following:

- Buddha Power Bowl (page 189)
- 5-ounce bacon cheeseburger (no bun) and a small green garden salad

DINNER

Choose one of the following:

- Salisbury Steaks with Rosemary-Buttered Mushrooms and Fresh Tomato Salad (page 183)
- 1 serving of Goat Cheese and Olive–Stuffed Chicken Breasts with Balsamic-Buttered Kale (see page 161)
- 6 ounces grilled or baked chicken breast or a 6-ounce grilled steak, your choice of cut

SNACKS

Choose two of the following to consume anytime of the day (but not consecutively and not within an hour before or after eating a meal):

- Keto peanut butter cookies (store-bought, 150-calorie serving)
- 10 organic seaweed snacks

- Keto protein bar (store-bought, 150-calorie serving)
- Keto tortilla chips (store-bought, 150-calorie serving)
- Pork rinds/cracklins (store-bought, 150-calorie serving)

EXERCISE

AM

Twenty-minute HIIT session. Don't eat anything until an hour after your workout.

MOVING ON

You've completed the six weeks and the big question is: What do you do next? Well, there is no one answer for everyone, since people have different goals, different demands on them, and different resources with which to reach those goals. The first thing I recommend for everyone, however, is to do another round of the program, even if you've hit your weight-loss goal. For those who don't need to lose any more weight, don't worry. You won't lose more weight if you don't need to. The purpose of doing a second cycle is to give your body another lap around the track, so that it can feel comfortable with improved metabolic flexibility and the lessons learned, and to help the adaptations you've made become more sustainable. Not only will you find that the second cycle is easier to do, but you will also be able to implement strategies you developed during the first cycle to make the plan work for you even better.

Whether or not you decide to do another cycle, the question remains: What is the long-term plan to maintain the results you've achieved? Once again, there is no one answer that applies to everyone. However, going back to your previous way of eating and moving will certainly deplete the gains you've made to improve your metabolic flexibility and lose weight. Going forward, even if you don't follow the plan specifically, think about alternating your weekly regimens, similar to what you did during weeks 3 to 6 on the plan. Divide your weeks up between carb-friendly days and a stretch of keto-friendly days. This pattern should keep your body challenged to continue efficiently burning whatever fuels are available. It's also important to monitor yourself for the signs of metabolic inflexibility described on page 10. If you are noticing two or more of these signs, earnestly re-engage with the plan. You don't need to do weeks 1 and 2 and can go straight to the last four weeks.

While all components of the plan are important for continued success, be mindful that the fasting and exercise strategies should become a fixed part of your regimen regardless of what you eat. You can mix it up by following the different fasting methods, but do your best to stick to whichever one you are currently following, as this will keep your metabolic flexibility tuned up. Continue doing fasted workouts at least a couple of times a week and at least two 20-minute resistance/strength training sessions per week. Taking these measures will keep you tuned up and prevent your body from straying too far from the new set point you've established since completing the plan.

Most important, remember two things: life is short, and no one is perfect. Don't be too hard on yourself or obsess over the small things. Your weight is going to fluctuate—everyone's does. Your goal is to avoid major fluctuations and keep the variance to less than 10 pounds. You won't always make the perfect dietary choice or exercise with the intensity or frequency that you want. That's not a problem. This is a long game and it's all about balance. Making better choices 70 percent of the time is more than enough to keep you in the range of where you want to be and will allow you to avoid feeling guilty about not being perfect or occasionally choosing to do your own thing when the plan says you should be doing something else. The plan is a blueprint, but you are the builder and interior designer. The final specifications are for you and you alone to decide. Carpe diem!

9

MET FLEX RECIPES

The following recipes will give you some new ideas for meals that you might not have tried before or a new take on some old recipes. They are low-carb or keto-friendly recipes. Be creative within the guidelines of the plan and pay close attention to the servings that the recipes yield, as well as how many servings you consume. You can alter the ingredient quantities to increase or decrease the number of servings you cook. Most important, have fun, keep an open mind, and enjoy the adventure of expanding your palate!

MEALS ▪ 135

SNACKS ▪ 201

SMOOTHIES ▪ 213

MEALS

CHIVE AND GRUYÈRE FRITTATA WITH CRAB AND AVOCADO

SERVES 4

8 ounces fresh crabmeat

2 teaspoons fresh lemon juice

2 teaspoons plus ¼ cup chopped fresh chives or finely chopped scallion greens

Kosher salt and freshly ground black pepper

10 large eggs

4 ounces Gruyère cheese, shredded (about 1 cup)

2 tablespoons grapeseed or sunflower oil

2 ripe avocados, pitted, peeled, and very thinly sliced

Preheat the oven to 425°F with a rack positioned in the center.

In a small bowl, gently toss the crabmeat with the lemon juice, 2 teaspoons chives, and a pinch of black pepper until combined. Set aside.

In a large bowl, whisk the eggs with ¼ cup chives, ½ teaspoon salt, and ¼ teaspoon black pepper until combined. Add ¾ of the cheese and combine.

Heat the oil in an oven-safe 12-inch nonstick skillet over medium heat until rippling. Pour in the egg mixture, swirling the pan to evenly distribute the eggs, and cook, without stirring, until the eggs are set around the edges, 4 to 5 minutes. Use a rubber spatula to release any of the edges that are stuck to the pan. Scatter the remaining cheese over the surface of the eggs and transfer the pan to the oven. Bake until the eggs are set on the surface and the cheese on top is melted and beginning to brown, 8 to 10 minutes.

Remove the pan from the oven (be sure to leave the hot pad or towel on the handle to prevent burns) and arrange the avocado slices evenly over the top of the frittata. Scatter the crab over the avocado and let the frittata stand for 10 minutes to cool briefly.

Slide the frittata onto a cutting board or plate and cut into wedges to serve.

CRUSTLESS BACON, ZUCCHINI, AND PEPPER JACK QUICHE

8 ounces thick-cut, no-sugar-added bacon, chopped

1 small yellow onion, chopped

1 clove garlic, minced

1 medium zucchini, quartered lengthwise and chopped into ¼-inch pieces

Kosher salt and freshly ground black pepper

8 large eggs

½ cup heavy cream or half-and-half

8 ounces pepper jack cheese, grated and divided

Hot sauce and sour cream, for serving (optional)

Preheat the oven to 350°F with the rack in the center position. Grease an 8-inch-square glass baking dish with cooking spray. Set a colander inside a larger bowl.

In a 12-inch skillet over medium heat, cook the bacon, stirring frequently, until crisp, 8 to 10 minutes. Using a slotted spoon, transfer the bacon to a large bowl. Add the onion and garlic to the skillet and cook, stirring, until softened, 5 to 6 minutes. Add the zucchini, ½ teaspoon salt, and ¼ teaspoon black pepper and cook, stirring often, until the zucchini has softened but still holds its shape, about 5 minutes. Pour the zucchini-onion mixture into the colander, spreading it out to drain, and cool briefly.

Add the eggs and cream to the bacon in the large bowl, along with ½ teaspoon salt, and whisk until combined. With a rubber spatula, fold the drained, cooled zucchini mixture into the eggs until evenly combined. Add ¾ of the grated cheese and mix well. Transfer to the baking dish and scatter the remaining cheese over the top. Bake until the eggs are set and the cheese is bubbly and beginning to brown, 30 to 40 minutes.

Cool for at least 10 minutes before slicing and serving with hot sauce and sour cream on the side.

KETO PANCAKES

2 PANCAKES PER SERVING

1 cup almond flour

1 teaspoon sweetener of your choice (such as monk fruit, yacón syrup, or stevia)

1 teaspoon baking powder

2 large eggs

1 teaspoon vanilla extract

⅓ cup almond or coconut milk

1 teaspoon coconut oil, melted

Low-carb syrup, for serving

In a small bowl, mix the flour, sweetener, and baking powder.

In a large bowl, whisk together the eggs, vanilla, milk, and coconut oil until combined.

Slowly fold the dry ingredients into the wet ingredients until fully combined.

Grease a large nonstick pan and place over medium heat. Pour the batter into the pan, approximately ⅓ cup at a time, to make 4 pancakes. Flip when edges begin to bubble. Cook for another couple of minutes, then serve hot with 1 tablespoon low-carb syrup.

BANANA NUT MUFFINS

SERVES 5

¾ cup almond flour

1 teaspoon baking powder

1 tablespoon ground flax

¼ teaspoon ground cinnamon

3 tablespoons butter, softened, plus more for greasing the pan

1 egg

¼ cup sweetener (such as organic stevia or monk fruit)

1 teaspoon vanilla extract

1 large banana, mashed (about ⅓ cup)

¼ cup unsweetened almond milk

¼ cup sour cream

½ cup walnuts, chopped

Preheat the oven to 350°F and lightly grease a muffin pan with butter or cooking spray.

In a large bowl, combine the almond flour, baking powder, flax, and cinnamon.

In a separate bowl, cream the butter, egg, sweetener, and vanilla.

Gently stir the banana, almond milk, sour cream, and walnuts into the egg mixture until fully combined. Add the wet ingredients to the dry ingredients and stir to combine.

Fill muffin cups about ¾ full, then bake for 20 to 25 minutes.

BACON EGG CUPS

SERVES 2

2 EGG CUPS PER SERVING

4 slices of thick center-cut bacon

1½ teaspoons extra-virgin olive oil

4 ounces mushrooms, sliced

1 clove garlic, minced

1 cup packed organic spinach

4 large eggs

1 teaspoon chopped chives

¼ cup unsweetened coconut or almond milk

Kosher salt and freshly ground black pepper

⅓ cup shredded cheddar or crumbled feta cheese

Preheat the oven to 400°F.

Arrange the bacon slices in a muffin pan, wrapping each around the interior edges of a cup. Bake for 10 minutes. Blot away any excessive grease in the cups after the bacon has cooked, leaving a little.

In a large skillet over medium-high heat, heat the olive oil and add the mushrooms and garlic. Cook until the mushrooms cook down and begin to brown, approximately 5 minutes. Add the spinach and cook for a few more minutes, or until the spinach wilts.

In a medium bowl, whisk together the eggs, chives, and milk. Season with salt and pepper.

Divide the veggies evenly between the four muffin cups. Pour the egg mixture into each cup and top with the cheese.

Bake for 15 minutes or until eggs are done to your preferred consistency. Let cool for a few minutes, then serve warm.

BREAKFAST BURRITO BOWL

SERVES 2

½ pound lean ground beef

1 tablespoon taco seasoning

½ head cauliflower, riced

4½ teaspoons chopped cilantro

¼ yellow onion, diced

Kosher salt and freshly ground black pepper

2 eggs

1 tablespoon butter, melted

2 tablespoons shredded cheese

In a large skillet over medium heat, brown the ground beef, then add ½ cup water and the taco seasoning. Bring to a boil, then reduce the heat and simmer for 2 to 3 minutes.

Once most of the water has cooked off, push the meat to the side of the skillet and add the riced cauliflower, cilantro, onion, and salt in the open space. Cook the cauliflower and onion for 5 minutes over low heat, then push the vegetables to the side to create space for the eggs. (If your skillet isn't large enough to accommodate cooking everything, you can scramble the eggs separately.)

Beat the eggs in a small bowl, then add them to the skillet and scramble with the butter and cheese. Once the eggs have cooked to your desired doneness, mix them with the other ingredients in the skillet. Separate into two bowls and season with salt and pepper to taste. Serve warm.

HAM, CHEESE, AND EGG ROLLS

SERVES 1

2 tablespoons grated
  Parmesan cheese

2 tablespoons shredded
  cheddar cheese

2 tablespoons shredded
  mozzarella cheese

1 egg

½ cup diced ham

Preheat the oven to 375°F. Line a medium baking sheet with parchment paper.

In a medium bowl, whisk together the Parmesan, shredded cheeses, and egg. Add in the diced ham and mix until just combined.

Pour the mixture onto the prepared baking sheet in three equal parts, forming round rolls.

Bake for 15 to 20 minutes, or until the cheese has fully melted and crusted slightly.

AVOCADO EGG BOATS

1 large avocado

2 large eggs

Kosher salt and freshly ground black pepper

2 tablespoons shredded cheddar cheese

1 teaspoon thinly sliced chives

1 tablespoon finely diced red bell pepper

Preheat the oven to 375°F.

Cut the avocado in half, remove the pit, and spoon out approximately 2 tablespoons of avocado flesh from the center, creating enough space to fit an egg.

Place the avocado halves cut side up in a baking dish. Fill each center with its own egg without breaking the yolk. Sprinkle with salt and black pepper.

Bake for 5 minutes, then sprinkle the shredded cheese on top. Continue to bake as needed to achieve desired doneness (an additional 5 to 6 minutes for soft, 7 to 8 minutes for medium, or 9 to 10 minutes for hard).

Sprinkle with the chives and bell pepper and serve warm.

SIMPLE EGG SALAD

SERVES 1

2 tablespoons mayonnaise

½ teaspoon mustard
(optional)

1 teaspoon freshly
squeezed lemon juice

2 tablespoons chopped
celery

1 tablespoon chopped
green onion

1 teaspoon chopped chives

1 large egg, hard-boiled,
peeled, and chopped

Kosher salt and freshly
ground black pepper

Pinch of curry powder or
paprika

In a medium bowl, whisk together the mayonnaise, mustard if desired, and lemon juice until smooth. Add the celery, onion, and chives and combine well.

In a separate bowl, using a fork, mash the hard-boiled egg slightly to your desired consistency.

Add the egg to the dressing, mixing well.

Season with salt and pepper to taste. Garnish with curry powder or paprika if desired.

BACON-STUFFED AVOCADOS

2 slices of bacon

1 medium avocado

¼ cup cherry tomatoes, halved

¼ cup chopped romaine lettuce

½ teaspoon mayonnaise

½ teaspoon lime juice

⅛ teaspoon garlic powder

Kosher salt and freshly ground black pepper

Cook the bacon in a skillet, being careful not to let it become too hard by overcooking it. You want it to maintain some flexibility. When done, set bacon on paper towel to drain.

Slice the avocado in half, remove the pit, and scoop out half of the flesh. Transfer the scooped-out avocado to a bowl and mash thoroughly.

Stir in the tomatoes, lettuce, mayonnaise, lime juice, garlic powder, salt, and pepper. Taste and adjust seasonings as desired.

Chop the bacon slices and add to the bowl.

Scoop the bacon-avocado mixture into the avocado halves.

ALMOND AND CHICHARRONES-CRUSTED PORK TENDERLOIN
WITH CHIPOTLE CAULIFLOWER SMASH

SERVES 4

¼ cup whole roasted unsalted almonds

1 cup snack chicharrones (fried pork rinds)

Kosher salt and freshly ground black pepper

1 pork tenderloin (about 1¼ pounds)

2 teaspoons Dijon mustard

1 head cauliflower (about 2 pounds), trimmed and coarsely chopped into 2-inch pieces

1 small canned chipotle in adobo, roughly chopped, plus 1 teaspoon adobo sauce from the can

3 tablespoons butter

1 teaspoon dried oregano

½ cup chopped fresh cilantro or scallions (optional)

Position the oven rack to the lower third position and preheat the oven to 425°F. Spray a baking sheet with cooking spray.

Put the almonds and chicharrones into a food storage bag and use a rolling pin or the bottom of a small saucepan to crush the nuts and pork rinds until finely ground. Lightly season the mixture with salt and pepper.

Pat the tenderloin dry with paper towels and season all over with salt and pepper. Using a pastry brush or spoon, evenly coat the pork all over with the Dijon mustard. Drop the meat into the nut mixture in the bag and press the nuts evenly into all sides of the meat until completely coated. Using tongs, remove the meat from the bag, shaking off the excess coating, and transfer to the greased baking sheet. Bake until an internal thermometer inserted into the thickest part of the meat registers 140°F, 20 to 25 minutes. Remove the meat from the oven and cover with aluminum foil to keep warm.

Meanwhile, put the cauliflower and chopped chipotle into a large saucepan and cover with water. Add 2 teaspoons salt, then bring to a boil over medium-high heat. Cover and reduce the heat to maintain a simmer, cooking until the cauliflower is very tender when pierced with a knife, 12 to 15 minutes. Drain the cauliflower and return it to the pan. Add the butter, adobo sauce, and oregano and, using a potato masher, mash until very smooth. Taste and season with salt and pepper.

Thinly slice the pork and serve with the cauliflower mash; garnish with the cilantro or scallions, if using.

GREEK PORK AND FETA MEATBALL LETTUCE WRAPS

SERVES 4

1 pound ground pork

½ cup crumbled feta

1 large egg

2 teaspoons chopped fresh oregano or 1 teaspoon dried

2 teaspoons chopped fresh dill or 1 teaspoon dried

¼ teaspoon garlic powder

1½ teaspoons kosher salt, plus more as needed

¾ teaspoon freshly ground black pepper, plus more as needed

3-inch section of English cucumber, plus thin slices for serving

2 tablespoons grapeseed or sunflower oil

½ cup whole-milk yogurt

2 teaspoons fresh lemon juice

8 butter lettuce or large romaine leaves

2 plum tomatoes, very thinly sliced

Mix the pork and feta in a large bowl with a rubber spatula to combine. In a small bowl, whisk together the egg, 2 tablespoons water, the oregano, dill, garlic powder, 1 teaspoon of the salt, and ½ teaspoon of the pepper until combined. Set aside for 10 minutes. Add the pork mixture to the egg mixture and stir until combined.

Meanwhile, grate the cucumber on the small holes of a box grater, then put it into a strainer set over a bowl. Sprinkle with the remaining ½ teaspoon salt and let stand while you cook the meatballs.

Divide the meat mixture into 24 balls, about 1 heaping table-spoon each. Roll them between your hands until smooth and transfer them to a plate.

In a 12-inch nonstick skillet, heat the oil over medium-high heat until rippling. Add the meatballs and cook without turning until lightly browned on the bottom, about 4 to 5 minutes. Using tongs, turn the meatballs, reduce the heat to medium, and continue cooking, turning frequently, until browned all over and an instant-read thermometer inserted into the center of a meatball reads 160°F, about 10 minutes total. Transfer the meatballs to a clean plate.

Using your hands, squeeze the grated cucumber firmly to drain as much liquid as possible from it and transfer it to a small bowl. Add the yogurt, lemon juice, and the remaining ¼ teaspoon black pepper and stir to combine. Taste and season with additional salt and pepper if desired.

Use cooking scissors to trim the lettuce leaves into bowls. Place the newly formed cups in a large bowl, cover with plastic wrap, and place in the refrigerator for 15 minutes before using.

To serve, fill the lettuce cups with tomato, cucumber slices, and meatballs and drizzle the yogurt sauce over the top.

PAN-SEARED PORK CHOPS

WITH ROMESCO BUTTER AND MANCHEGO BROCCOLI

SERVES 4

4 tablespoons butter, softened

¼ cup sliced almonds, toasted

3 tablespoons jarred roasted red peppers, diced, drained, and patted dry

2 teaspoons smoked paprika

1 clove garlic, smashed

2 teaspoons red wine vinegar

Kosher salt and freshly ground black pepper

4 bone-in pork chops (each about 8 ounces and 1 inch thick)

2 tablespoons extra-virgin olive oil

1 pound broccoli, trimmed and cut into florets

1 ounce Manchego cheese, shaved with a vegetable peeler

Put the butter, almonds, peppers, 1 teaspoon of the paprika, the garlic, vinegar, ½ teaspoon salt, and ¼ teaspoon pepper into a small food processor and puree until smooth. Transfer to a bowl.

In a small bowl, stir together the remaining 1 teaspoon smoked paprika, 1 teaspoon salt, and ½ teaspoon black pepper until combined. Pat the pork chops dry with a paper towel and season them on both sides with the spice mixture.

Heat 1 tablespoon of the oil in a 12-inch nonstick skillet over medium-high heat until rippling. Add 2 of the chops and cook, without moving, until golden brown on the bottom, about 4 to 5 minutes. Flip the chops, reduce the heat to medium, and cook until the chops are firm to the touch and register 135°F on an instant-read thermometer. Transfer the chops to a plate and cover with aluminum foil to keep warm. Wipe out the skillet with a paper towel and repeat with the remaining 1 tablespoon oil and 2 pork chops.

Meanwhile, fill a large saucepan one third with water, fit with a steamer basket, and bring to a simmer over medium-high heat. Add the broccoli, cover, and steam until crisp-tender (5 to 6 minutes). Transfer to a serving bowl; season lightly with salt and pepper.

To serve, dollop the Romesco butter over the warm chops and serve with the broccoli. Scatter the Manchego over the top.

ITALIAN SAUSAGE, SPINACH, AND CHEESE-STUFFED PORTOBELLO MUSHROOMS

SERVES 4

8 medium portobello mushrooms, stems and gills removed

2 tablespoons extra-virgin olive oil

Kosher salt and freshly ground black pepper

1 pound no-sugar-added sweet or hot Italian sausage, casings removed, or bulk sausages

4 oil-packed sun-dried tomatoes, drained and chopped

6 scallions, sliced, white and green parts separated

One 10-ounce box frozen chopped spinach, thawed and squeezed dry

½ cup shredded mozzarella (about 2 ounces)

½ cup shredded provolone or white cheddar cheese (about 2 ounces)

1 tablespoon balsamic vinegar

¼ cup chopped fresh basil or 1 tablespoon dried

Preheat the oven to 425°F. Line a rimmed baking sheet with aluminum foil.

Brush the mushrooms on both sides with the olive oil and season them lightly with salt and pepper. Place them on the baking sheet, stem side down, and roast for 10 minutes. Remove from the oven and cool.

Meanwhile, put the sausage, sun-dried tomatoes, and scallion whites in a nonstick skillet over medium-high heat and cook, breaking up the sausage with a spoon, until browned and no pink remains, about 10 minutes. Transfer the meat mixture to a medium bowl, add the spinach, and toss well to combine. Let come to room temperature. Then stir the cheeses and vinegar into the sausage until well combined. Add the basil and toss.

Turn the mushrooms stem side up. Using a large spoon, evenly stuff the mushroom cavities with the sausage and cheese mixture. Then bake the mushrooms until very hot and the cheese is bubbling and beginning to brown, about 12 to 14 minutes.

Serve the mushrooms with the scallion greens scattered over the top.

MASALA-DUSTED CHICKEN THIGHS
WITH GARLICKY BROWN
BUTTER SPINACH

SERVES 4

3 pounds bone-in, skin-on chicken thighs, trimmed

2 tablespoons extra-virgin olive oil

2 tablespoons garam masala spice blend

2 teaspoons kosher salt, plus more as needed

4 tablespoons butter

3 large cloves garlic, peeled and smashed with the side of a knife

¼ cup sliced almonds

2 large shallots, sliced

1 pound baby spinach

Preheat the oven to 450°F with the rack in the middle position. Grease a sheet pan with cooking spray.

Put the chicken thighs in a large bowl; drizzle the olive oil over the chicken and toss with tongs to coat. Sprinkle the garam masala and 2 teaspoons salt over the chicken, then toss the chicken with the tongs, distributing the spices evenly over the surface of the chicken. Arrange the thighs on the sheet pan, skin side up, and roast in the oven until browned and crisp and the chicken reaches an internal temperature of 175°F, about 35 minutes.

Meanwhile, put the butter, garlic, and almonds in a large skillet over medium heat. Cook, stirring frequently, until the almonds begin to lightly brown, 3 to 4 minutes. Using a slotted spoon, transfer the almonds to a plate. Continue cooking the garlic, stirring frequently, until deep golden brown, 2 to 3 minutes more. Remove the garlic and discard. Continue cooking the butter, swirling the pan, until it begins to turn a nutty golden brown. Add the shallots and cook, stirring frequently, until softened, about 2 minutes. Working in batches, add the spinach to the pan and toss with tongs until lightly wilted. Taste and season with salt.

To serve, divide the spinach among 4 plates. Top with the chicken thighs and sprinkle the toasted almonds over the top.

GOAT CHEESE AND OLIVE-STUFFED CHICKEN BREASTS

WITH BALSAMIC-BUTTERED KALE

SERVES 4

Four boneless, skinless chicken breasts (12 ounces each)

2 tablespoons extra-virgin olive oil

Kosher salt and freshly ground black pepper

4 ounces fresh goat cheese, at room temperature

¼ cup finely grated Parmesan or Romano cheese

⅓ cup pitted green olives, finely chopped

1 teaspoon chopped fresh rosemary or chives

½ cup balsamic vinegar

3 tablespoons butter

2 large shallots, sliced

2 bunches (about 2 pounds) of Lacinato kale, leaves stripped and coarsely chopped

Preheat the oven to 375°F with the rack in the middle position. Line a baking sheet with aluminum foil.

Using a sharp knife, cut a horizontal pocket into the side of each chicken breast, leaving the outer ½-inch edges attached. Brush the chicken with the oil and season both sides generously with salt and pepper.

In a medium bowl, use a rubber spatula to stir the goat cheese and Parmesan together until well combined. Add the olives and rosemary and mix well. Season with a generous pinch of black pepper and a bit of salt if desired. Using a large spoon, stuff ¼ of the cheese mixture into the pocket of each chicken breast and press on the breast lightly to evenly distribute the stuffing.

Transfer the chicken to the oven and bake until the chicken is cooked through, the juices run clear when pierced with a knife, and an instant-read thermometer inserted into the thickest part of a breast registers 160°F, about 25 minutes.

Meanwhile, put the balsamic vinegar in a small saucepan and simmer over medium heat until the liquid has reduced by about half and become syrupy, about 10 minutes. Remove from the heat.

Melt the butter in a 12-inch skillet over medium-high heat. Add the shallots and cook, stirring, until softened, 3 to 4 minutes. Add the kale in batches and toss with tongs until lightly wilted but not mushy. Season with salt and pepper.

To serve, divide the kale among 4 plates, place the chicken breasts on top of the kale, and drizzle the balsamic syrup over both.

COCONUT CHICKEN, CASHEW, AND ASPARAGUS STIR-FRY
WITH BUTTER-SOY CAULIFLOWER RICE

¼ cup low-sodium soy sauce

2 tablespoons unseasoned rice vinegar

1 teaspoon finely minced garlic (about 2 cloves)

1 tablespoon xanthan gum (optional)

Pinch of red chili flakes (optional)

2 pounds boneless, skinless chicken thighs, cut into 1-inch pieces

½ cup unsweetened coconut water

¼ cup coconut oil

1 pound asparagus, trimmed and sliced on the diagonal into 1-inch pieces

½ cup roasted cashews, roughly chopped

4 cups raw riced cauliflower

2 tablespoons butter

1 teaspoon fresh lime zest

Kosher salt and freshly ground black pepper

In a medium bowl, stir together 3 tablespoons of the soy sauce and the vinegar, garlic, xanthan gum, and chili flakes, if using. Add the chicken and stir to coat. Let stand for 10 minutes.

Set a fine strainer over a bowl and pour the chicken and marinade into it. Let stand for a couple of minutes, pressing on the chicken to remove as much liquid as possible. Whisk the coconut water into the marinade in the bowl.

Heat 2 tablespoons of the coconut oil in a 12-inch nonstick skillet over medium-high heat until rippling. Add the chicken in a single layer and cook, without turning, until golden brown on the bottom, 5 to 6 minutes. Stir with a silicone spatula, add the asparagus, and cook, stirring often, until the chicken is no longer pink, 3 to 4 minutes. Add the marinade mixture and cashews and cook, stirring, another 3 to 4 minutes, until the liquid is simmering, the chicken is cooked through, and the sauce begins to thicken. Transfer to a serving bowl and cover to keep warm.

Wipe the skillet clean with a paper towel. Add the remaining coconut oil over medium-high heat and, when rippling, add the cauliflower. Cook, stirring often, until the cauliflower rice is tender-crisp and beginning to brown, 4 to 5 minutes. Add the butter and remaining 1 tablespoon soy sauce and cook, stirring, until the butter is melted and the cauliflower rice is evenly coated. Remove from heat and stir in the lime zest. Taste and season with salt and pepper.

Serve the cauliflower rice with the chicken stir-fry spooned over the top.

MEDITERRANEAN CHICKEN SKEWERS

WITH SHAVED CARROT AND WALNUT SALAD

SERVES 4

3 tablespoons fresh lemon juice

¼ cup extra-virgin olive oil

1 tablespoon dried oregano

1 teaspoon ground cumin

1 teaspoon ground coriander

Kosher salt and freshly ground black pepper

1½ pounds boneless, skinless chicken thighs, cut into 1-inch-wide strips

4 large carrots (about 12 ounces)

2 tablespoons red wine vinegar

½ cup fresh mint leaves, roughly torn

½ cup toasted walnuts, roughly chopped

Preheat the broiler with the rack 4 to 6 inches from the element. Line a baking sheet with aluminum foil.

In a medium bowl, whisk together the lemon juice, 2 tablespoons of the olive oil, the dried oregano, cumin, coriander, 1 teaspoon salt, and ½ teaspoon pepper until combined. Add the chicken and toss to combine. Let stand for 10 to 15 minutes.

Using a vegetable peeler, shave the carrots lengthwise, turning as you pull strips off the carrots, until you reach the cores.

Put the carrot strips in a large bowl. Toss with the remaining 2 tablespoons olive oil, vinegar, ½ teaspoon salt, and ¼ teaspoon pepper. Set aside at room temperature to allow the carrots to soften.

Thread the chicken onto 8 long metal grilling skewers and arrange them in a single layer on the baking sheet. Broil until the chicken is golden brown, crisp at the edges, and cooked through, 12 to 14 minutes. Turn the skewers once during cooking. Remove from the oven and cool briefly before serving.

Add the mint leaves and walnuts to the carrots, toss to combine, and transfer to a large platter. Serve the chicken skewers resting on the carrot salad.

SPICY CHICKEN AND PEANUT LETTUCE WRAPS WITH CUCUMBER

SERVES 4

- 2 tablespoons fresh lime juice
- 1 tablespoon fish sauce or soy sauce
- 1 tablespoon unseasoned rice vinegar
- ½ teaspoon each kosher salt and freshly ground black pepper
- 3 tablespoons grapeseed, sunflower, or coconut oil
- 2 large shallots, sliced into thin rings
- 1 large Fresno or red jalapeño chile, stemmed, seeded, and minced
- 1 pound ground chicken or turkey
- ⅓ cup roasted peanuts, chopped
- ½ cup fresh mint leaves, chopped
- 8 large romaine lettuce leaves (about 2 hearts)
- ½ English cucumber, halved lengthwise and thinly sliced on the diagonal

In a small bowl, whisk together the lime juice, fish sauce, vinegar, salt, and pepper until combined.

Heat the oil in a 12-inch nonstick skillet over medium-high heat until rippling. Add the shallots and chile and cook, stirring, until softened, 3 to 4 minutes. Add the chicken and cook, breaking the meat up into small bits with a spatula, until completely cooked through and no pink remains, 5 to 6 minutes.

Add the lime juice mixture to the skillet and cook until the liquid is simmering and coats the meat. Remove from heat and stir in the peanuts and mint leaves.

To serve, line the romaine leaves with cucumber slices and spoon the chicken mixture over the top.

CHICKEN BROCCOLI CASSEROLE

SERVES 4

- ½ pound broccoli, cut into florets
- 2 cups shredded cooked chicken
- 6 ounces cream cheese
- 1 cup grated cheddar cheese
- ½ cup almond milk
- 1 tablespoon Dijon mustard
- 1 teaspoon garlic powder
- ¼ teaspoon salt
- ¼ teaspoon ground black pepper
- ¼ cup chopped fresh basil
- ¼ cup mayonnaise
- ¼ cup grated Parmesan cheese

Preheat the oven to 350°F.

Place broccoli florets in a medium pot of water over high heat and boil until al dente. Drain well, then add to a large bowl with the chicken.

In a small saucepan, simmer cream cheese, cheddar cheese, almond milk, mustard, garlic powder, salt, and pepper over low heat. Whisk vigorously until the sauce has a smooth consistency.

Pour the warm sauce over the broccoli and chicken mixture, add basil and mayonnaise, and mix well.

Transfer entire mixture to a casserole dish and sprinkle the Parmesan cheese over the top.

Bake for 15 to 20 minutes, or until the entire casserole is warmed through and the cheese has slightly browned. Serve warm.

ROASTED CITRUS-MISO SALMON AND GREEN BEANS

SERVES 4

3 tablespoons white miso

2 tablespoons grapeseed or sunflower oil

2 tablespoons fresh orange juice

1 tablespoon fresh lime juice, plus wedges for serving

2 teaspoons low-sodium soy sauce

1 pound green beans, trimmed

4 skin-on center-cut salmon fillets (about 6 ounces each)

1 teaspoon sesame seeds, toasted

Preheat the oven to 450°F with the rack in the middle position. Grease a heavy baking sheet with cooking spray.

In a small bowl, whisk together the miso, oil, orange and lime juices, and soy sauce until combined. Put the green beans in a large bowl, add 1 tablespoon of the miso mixture, and toss the beans to coat them well.

Evenly brush the salmon (top and sides) with the remaining miso mixture and let stand at room temperature for about 10 minutes.

Evenly spread the green beans on the baking sheet and transfer to the oven. Roast for 6 minutes until sizzling and beginning to brown. Remove the pan from the oven and carefully stir the beans. Using tongs, transfer the salmon to the baking sheet, resting the fillets directly on top of the beans. Return the pan to the oven and roast until the salmon is firm to the touch and an instant-read thermometer registers 120°F at the thickest point, about 10 minutes.

Remove the pan from the oven and let stand for about 10 minutes to cool. Serve the salmon and green beans sprinkled with sesame seeds and with lime wedges for squeezing on the side.

CURRIED COCONUT COD, SHRIMP, AND FENNEL STEW

SERVES 4

2 tablespoons grapeseed or sunflower oil

1 large fennel bulb, trimmed, cored, and very thinly sliced

2 cloves garlic, thinly sliced

½ teaspoon each kosher salt and freshly ground black pepper, plus more as needed

One 8-ounce bottle of clam juice

1 serrano or small jalapeño pepper, stemmed, seeded, and halved lengthwise

One 14-ounce can unsweetened coconut milk

1 large ripe tomato (about 12 ounces), cored, seeded, and chopped

1-pound fresh cod fillet, cut into 2-inch pieces

12 ounces medium peeled shrimp, tails removed

2 teaspoons fresh lime juice, plus wedges for serving

½ cup finely chopped fresh basil or parsley

In a deep 12-inch skillet or Dutch oven, heat the oil over medium heat until shimmering. Add the fennel, garlic, salt, and pepper, and cook, stirring frequently, until very soft, about 10 to 12 minutes.

Add the clam juice and serrano pepper, bring to a simmer, and cook for 5 minutes. Add the coconut milk and chopped tomato, reduce the heat to medium-low, and cook at a simmer until the tomato just begins to break down, about 5 to 6 minutes. Stir in the cod and shrimp and cook, gently stirring, until the liquid begins to simmer again, about 2 minutes. Remove the pan from the heat, cover, and let stand until the fish and shrimp are cooked through in the residual heat, about 8 to 10 minutes.

Remove the lid, stir the stew gently, remove the serrano pepper, and stir in the lime juice and basil. Serve in four bowls, with lime wedges on the side for squeezing.

CREAMY GARLIC PARMESAN ZUCCHINI NOODLES WITH SHRIMP

SERVES 4

1 cup heavy cream

3 large cloves garlic, smashed

1 teaspoon kosher salt, plus more as needed

½ teaspoon freshly ground black pepper, plus more as needed

1 pound large shrimp, peeled and tails removed

½ cup grated Parmesan, plus more for serving

12 ounces fresh zucchini or yellow squash noodles (spiralized squash)

½ cup chopped fresh basil or parsley

In a 12-inch skillet over medium-high heat, bring the cream and garlic to a simmer. Reduce the heat to medium and continue to simmer until the liquid thickens slightly, 5 to 6 minutes. Add the salt, pepper, and shrimp, stirring, until the shrimp begin to turn pink, 3 to 4 minutes.

Stir in the Parmesan cheese and zucchini noodles and cook, tossing gently, until the shrimp is cooked through and the noodles are lightly cooked but still firm, about 2 minutes. Taste the sauce and season with salt and pepper. Remove the garlic cloves and discard.

Remove from the heat and stir in the basil. Serve the "pasta" with additional cheese grated over the top.

CRISPY ROASTED
CAULIFLOWER STEAKS
WITH ZUCCHINI "GHANOUSH"

SERVES 4

2 heads cauliflower (about 2 pounds each), leaves trimmed but with the core left intact

1 tablespoon sweet paprika, plus more to serve

Kosher salt and freshly ground black pepper

Extra-virgin olive oil

2 cloves garlic, chopped

1 pound zucchini, stemmed, quartered lengthwise, and cut into small cubes

¼ cup tahini

¼ cup whole-milk Greek yogurt

2 tablespoons fresh lemon juice

2 scallions, thinly sliced (optional)

Preheat the oven to 450°F with a rack in the middle position. Grease a rimmed baking sheet with cooking spray.

Set the cauliflower heads upright on a cutting board. Using a sharp knife, cut two 1-inch-wide slabs out of the center of each cauliflower and place the cauliflower steaks on the baking sheet in a single layer. Coarsely chop the remaining cauliflower and set aside.

In a small bowl, stir together the paprika, 1 teaspoon salt, and ½ teaspoon pepper until combined. Drizzle about 2 tablespoons olive oil over the cauliflower steaks, then use a brush to coat the surfaces evenly. Flip the steaks and brush the other side. Evenly sprinkle the paprika mixture over the cauliflower. Transfer to the oven and bake until the cauliflower steaks are tender when pierced with a knife and crispy brown at the edges, about 30 to 35 minutes. Flip them once halfway through.

Meanwhile, heat 1 tablespoon oil in a 12-inch skillet over medium-high heat. Add the chopped cauliflower and season it lightly with salt and pepper. Cook, stirring, until the cauliflower begins to brown at the edges, about 5 minutes. Pour ¼ cup water into the skillet, cover, and cook until the cauliflower is completely tender and falling apart, about 10 minutes. Transfer to a medium bowl.

Return the pan to the stove and heat 1 tablespoon oil over medium heat. Add the garlic and zucchini, season lightly with a pinch of salt and pepper, stir well, cover the pan, and cook, stirring occasionally, until the zucchini is very soft and beginning to break down, about 5 minutes. Remove the lid and continue cooking until the liquid in the pan evaporates, about 3 to 4 minutes longer.

While the zucchini cooks, mash the cooked cauliflower pieces with a potato masher until they match the consistency of mashed potatoes. Add the tahini, yogurt, and lemon juice and mix well. Fold the cooked zucchini into the mixture along with ½ teaspoon each salt and pepper. Toss lightly to evenly combine.

To serve, put the cauliflower steaks on plates and scoop the zucchini mixture on top of each steak. Sprinkle generously with paprika and garnish with the scallions, if using.

THREE-CHEESE EGGPLANT AND ASPARAGUS ROLLATINI WITH PESTO

SERVES 4

2 medium globe eggplant (about 1 pound each)

3 tablespoons extra-virgin olive oil

Kosher salt and freshly ground black pepper

1 pound medium asparagus, trimmed and halved crosswise

8 ounces whole-milk mozzarella cheese, shredded

2 ounces provolone or Asiago cheese, shredded

¼ cup grated Parmesan cheese

1 teaspoon dried oregano

1 cup prepared pesto

Toasted pine nuts, for garnish (optional)

Preheat the oven to 425°F with two racks in the upper and lower third positions.

Thinly slice the eggplant crosswise into ¼-inch-wide slices and arrange them on a baking sheet in a single layer. Brush both sides of the slices with 2 tablespoons of the olive oil and season them generously with salt and pepper. Put the asparagus in a 9 × 13-inch baking dish, toss with the remaining 1 tablespoon oil, and season with salt and pepper. Put the eggplant on the lower rack and the asparagus on the upper rack and roast until the eggplant is softened but not brown, about

10 minutes. Remove the vegetables from the oven and let stand until cool enough to handle.

Meanwhile, in a medium bowl, toss the cheeses and oregano together until combined. Reserve about ½ cup of the mixture. Arrange the cooled eggplant on a work surface and place 2 asparagus spears in the center of each slice. Evenly spread the cheese mixture over the top of each eggplant slice and tightly roll them into cylinders. Arrange the vegetable rolls in the baking dish in a single layer.

Spoon the pesto evenly over the tops of the rolls and scatter the reserved cheese mixture over the top. Bake until the sauce is bubbling and the cheese is melted and beginning to brown on top, 12 to 15 minutes.

Remove the dish from the oven and let stand for about 10 minutes to cool. Serve the rollatini sprinkled with pine nuts, if using.

PHILLY CHEESE STEAK AND ROASTED TOMATO MELTS

2 large beefsteak tomatoes, each cut into 4 thick slices (about ½ inch thick)

2 tablespoons extra-virgin olive oil

Kosher salt and freshly ground black pepper

1 medium yellow onion, sliced

1 red bell pepper, very thinly sliced

1 pound shaved beef

2 tablespoons butter

8 slices of provolone cheese, roughly chopped, or 8 ounces shredded provolone

Preheat the broiler with the rack positioned 6 inches from the element. Place a metal cooling rack on a rimmed baking sheet and spray with cooking spray.

Arrange the tomatoes in a single layer on top of the rack in the pan, drizzle 1 tablespoon oil over the slices, and season with ½ teaspoon each salt and pepper. Place the pan under the broiler and cook until the tomatoes are bubbling and beginning to char around the edges, 6 to 8 minutes. Remove the pan from the oven, but leave the broiler on.

Heat the remaining 1 tablespoon oil in a 12-inch nonstick skillet over medium-high heat until rippling. Add the onion, bell pepper, and ½ teaspoon each salt and pepper and cook, stirring frequently, until the onion is completely soft and beginning to brown, 8 to 10 minutes. Transfer the vegetables to a large bowl.

Return the pan to medium-high heat and, when very hot, add the shaved steak in an even layer. Season lightly with salt and pepper and cook, without stirring, until the meat is browned on the bottom but still pink. Transfer the meat to the bowl with the vegetables, add the butter, and stir well to combine. Add half of the chopped cheese and stir quickly to combine.

Using a large spoon, divide the meat mixture evenly among the tomato slices, mounding the filling on top of each slice. Scatter the remaining chopped cheese evenly over the top of each covered tomato slice. Broil until the mixture is sizzling and hot and the cheese on top is melted and beginning to brown, about 2 to 3 minutes.

Cool for 5 minutes before serving.

CHILI-RUBBED FLANK STEAK
WITH CHIPOTLE BUTTER AND
CHARRED LIME BROCCOLI

SERVES 4

1-pound flank steak

1 teaspoon kosher salt,
plus more as needed

½ teaspoon freshly ground
black pepper, plus more
as needed

1 teaspoon ground cumin

1 teaspoon ground
coriander

½ teaspoon chili powder
or chipotle powder

¼ cup extra-virgin olive oil

4 tablespoons butter,
softened

1 canned chipotle in adobo
sauce, finely minced

1 pound broccoli crowns,
trimmed and cut into
florets

Finely grated zest of 1 lime,
plus wedges for serving

½ cup chopped fresh
cilantro leaves, for
garnish (optional)

Preheat the oven to 475°F.

Pat the steak dry with paper towels. In a small bowl, stir together 1 tablespoon salt, ½ teaspoon pepper, cumin, coriander, and chili powder until combined. Reserve 1 teaspoon of the spice mixture; set aside. Brush the steak on both sides with 1 tablespoon olive oil and evenly sprinkle the rest of the spice mixture on both sides, rubbing it into the meat. Let stand for 10 minutes.

In a small bowl, mash the butter with the minced chipotle and a pinch of salt until combined. Set aside.

Scatter the broccoli on a heavy baking sheet, drizzle with 1 tablespoon olive oil, sprinkle the reserved spice mixture over it, and toss to coat well. Roast in the oven until charred and crisp at the edges, 10 to 12 minutes, stirring once halfway through. Remove from the oven and toss the hot broccoli with the lime zest. Season with additional salt and pepper, if needed.

Heat the remaining 2 tablespoons oil in a skillet over medium-high heat. Add the steak and cook, without moving, until well browned on the bottom, 4 to 5 minutes. Flip the steak, reduce the heat to medium, and continue cooking until the steak is firm to the touch and, for medium-rare steak, registers 125°F, about 3 to 4 minutes more. Transfer the steak to a plate and let stand for 10 minutes.

Meanwhile, remove the pan from the heat and add the chipotle butter, stirring and scraping up any browned bits as the butter melts; leave the sauce in the pan.

Pour any of the juices the steak has released back into the skillet with the butter sauce. Thinly slice the steak across the grain and return it to the plate. Drizzle the butter sauce over the steak, sprinkle with cilantro (if using), and serve with the broccoli and lime wedges for squeezing.

SALISBURY STEAKS
WITH ROSEMARY-BUTTERED MUSHROOMS AND FRESH TOMATO SALAD

SERVES 4

1 pound ground beef, preferably 80 percent lean

1 small sweet onion, finely chopped

2 large eggs, beaten

1 tablespoon Worcestershire sauce or soy sauce

Kosher salt and freshly ground black pepper

¼ cup finely crushed low-carb crackers

2 tablespoons extra-virgin olive oil, plus more as needed

4 tablespoons butter

1 pound cremini mushrooms, trimmed and thinly sliced

1 tablespoon chopped fresh rosemary or 1½ teaspoons dried

1 teaspoon finely minced fresh ginger or ½ teaspoon dried

1 pound very ripe tomatoes, preferably heirloom, thinly sliced

2 teaspoons red wine vinegar

½ cup fresh basil leaves, torn, or 2 teaspoons dried basil

Put the beef and onion in a medium bowl. In a separate small bowl, whisk the eggs, Worcestershire (or soy), 2 teaspoons salt, and 1 teaspoon black pepper until combined. Add the crushed crackers, stir to combine, and let stand to soften for about 5 minutes. Add the egg mixture to the beef and, using your hands, combine the ingredients well. Divide the mixture into 4 equal portions and form them into patties about ½ inch thick.

Heat the oil in a nonstick skillet over medium-high heat until rippling. Add the beef patties to the pan and cook until well browned on the bottoms, 4 to 5 minutes. Flip the patties, reduce the heat to medium, and continue cooking until the burgers are firm to the touch and the internal temperature is 130°F in the center, 4 to 5 minutes more. Transfer the patties to a plate and cover with aluminum foil to keep warm.

Add the butter, mushrooms, rosemary, ginger, and a generous pinch of salt and pepper to the pan and cook over medium-high heat, stirring and scraping the browned bits off the pan with a rubber spatula, until the mushrooms are soft, beginning to brown, and have released all of their liquid, 8 to 10 minutes.

To serve, add any juices the patties have released to the mushrooms and stir them. Divide the tomatoes among 4 plates, then drizzle the vinegar and some olive oil over them. Season the tomatoes with salt and pepper, scatter the basil over them, and serve the Salisbury steaks on top of the tomatoes covered with the mushrooms.

STEAK TIP CACCIATORE
WITH CAULIFLOWER RICE

SERVES 4

1 pound steak tips, cut into 1-inch pieces

Kosher salt and freshly ground black pepper

2 tablespoons olive oil

1 medium onion, sliced

3 cloves garlic, thinly sliced

8 ounces cremini mushrooms, trimmed and quartered

1 small red bell pepper, stemmed, seeded, and chopped into 1-inch pieces

1 small green bell pepper, stemmed, seeded, and chopped into 1-inch pieces

One 14-ounce can no-sugar-added tomato puree

Pinch of red chili flakes

4 cups raw riced cauliflower

3 tablespoons butter

Handful of fresh basil leaves, torn, or 1 teaspoon dried basil or Italian seasoning

Season the steak all over with 2 teaspoons salt and ½ teaspoon black pepper.

Heat the oil in a 12-inch nonstick skillet over medium-high heat until rippling. Add the steak tips in a single layer and cook, without stirring, until golden on the bottom, 2 to 3 minutes. Stir and continue cooking until the beef is no longer pink on the surface. Transfer the beef to a plate.

Add the onion, garlic, mushrooms, and ½ teaspoon each salt and pepper to the skillet and cook, stirring occasionally, until the onion and mushrooms are soft and beginning to brown, 6 to 8 minutes. Add the chopped peppers and continue to cook until peppers are softened, about 5 minutes. Stir in the tomato puree and red chili flakes and bring to a simmer. Cover the pan, lower the heat to medium, and cook until the vegetables are very soft, 6 to 8 minutes.

Meanwhile, put the cauliflower rice in a microwaveable bowl with 1 tablespoon water, ½ teaspoon salt, and ¼ teaspoon black pepper and cover with a lid. Cook on high for 4 minutes. Remove the bowl from the microwave, carefully remove the lid, and stir in the butter until melted.

When the peppers in the skillet are soft, add the beef tips with their juices and cook, stirring, until the meat is warmed through but still pink in the center, about 2 minutes. Remove from the heat and stir in the basil leaves or dried seasoning and let stand for about 5 minutes before serving.

Serve the steak mixture over the hot buttered cauliflower rice.

ENCHILADA BOWL

1 tablespoon extra-virgin olive oil

½ cup chopped onion

½ bell pepper, chopped

2 ounces green chiles, diced

½ teaspoon sea salt

¼ teaspoon pepper

2 tablespoons taco seasoning

1½ cups shredded cooked chicken

½ cup cottage cheese

¾ cup shredded cheddar cheese

6 ounces red enchilada sauce

2 cups cooked cauliflower rice

Preheat the oven to 400°F.

Heat the olive oil in a large oven-safe pan over medium heat.

Add the chopped onion and pepper and sauté until soft, about 10 minutes.

Reduce the heat to low, then stir in the diced green chiles, ¼ cup water, salt, pepper, and taco seasoning. Continue stirring until the taco seasoning dissolves.

Add the chicken, cottage cheese, half of the cheddar cheese, and the red enchilada sauce. Stir until all ingredients are well combined.

Sprinkle the remaining cheddar cheese over the top.

Bake for 10 to 15 minutes, or until the cheese starts to brown around the edges.

Serve over the cauliflower rice. Enjoy!

BUDDHA POWER BOWL

4 cups spinach

1 tablespoon extra-virgin
  olive oil

1 cup cauliflower rice

Sea salt and freshly
  cracked black pepper

1 large avocado, pitted,
  peeled, and sliced

1 red radish

1 medium carrot

½ cup shredded red
  cabbage

½ cup cooked chickpeas

1 tablespoon sesame seeds

Freshly squeezed juice
  from 1 large lemon

Tahini sauce, for serving

Divide the spinach between two bowls.

Heat the olive oil in a skillet over high heat, then add the cauliflower rice and sauté for a few minutes. Lightly season with salt and pepper.

Divide the cauliflower rice between the bowls and top each one with half the avocado slices.

Slice the radish into thin rounds and use a vegetable peeler to peel the carrot into ribbons. In a separate bowl, toss the cabbage, radish slices, chickpeas, sesame seeds, and carrots in the lemon juice. Divide and add to each bowl.

Season with salt and pepper and serve with the tahini sauce.

DECONSTRUCTED EGG ROLL

SERVES 2

1 tablespoon extra-virgin olive oil, plus more for browning

½ pound ground beef or pork

½ teaspoon minced garlic

6 ounces shredded cabbage

2 tablespoons reduced-sodium soy sauce

1 egg, beaten

2 teaspoons hot sauce, plus more as needed

1 tablespoon sesame oil

Pour a small amount of olive oil into a large skillet over medium heat and brown the beef or pork all the way through, about 8 to 10 minutes.

Drain the meat, then add the garlic, making sure not to overcook it, about 1 minute.

Add the cabbage and soy sauce and sauté until tender.

Move everything to the side of the skillet and make room to scramble the egg. Stir the hot sauce into the egg while it is cooking.

Once the egg has cooked, divide the ingredients into equal portions and assemble in two bowls or on two plates. Drizzle with the sesame oil and add more hot sauce and soy sauce if desired.

SALMON AVOCADO POWER BOWL

SERVES 2

The Bowl

6 ounces salmon, skin removed

½ teaspoon salt

2 cups baby spinach, washed and dried

1 medium cucumber, peeled and diced

1 cup cauliflower florets, cooked

½ large avocado, pitted, peeled, and sliced

1 cup cherry tomatoes, halved

½ cup crumbled feta cheese

1 small radish, sliced

Creamy Dill Dressing

⅓ cup mayonnaise

2 tablespoons extra-virgin olive oil

½ cup full-fat Greek yogurt

1 teaspoon lemon zest

1 tablespoon lemon juice

1 teaspoon Dijon mustard

1 clove garlic, minced

¼ cup chopped fresh dill

Kosher salt and freshly ground black pepper

Preheat the oven to 350°F. Line a baking dish with aluminum foil.

Add all dressing ingredients to a small bowl and whisk together until blended.

Season the salmon with the salt, then place in the prepared baking dish and bake until the salmon reaches the desired temperature (about 6 minutes for medium rare and 11 minutes for medium). Once cool, cut the salmon into even chunks.

Divide the salmon, spinach, cucumber, cauliflower, avocado, and tomatoes between two bowls. Scatter the feta cheese and radish slices on top and drizzle with the creamy dill dressing.

MEATBALL BOWL

Meatballs

½ pound lean ground beef

¼ cup keto breadcrumbs

2 teaspoons soy sauce

½ teaspoon sriracha

¼ cup diced white onion

¼ teaspoon kosher salt

¼ teaspoon freshly ground black pepper

The Bowl

1 medium cucumber, peeled and chopped

2 tablespoons rice wine vinegar

1 teaspoon red chili flakes (optional)

2 cups cauliflower rice, cooked

Sauce

⅓ cup mayonnaise

½ teaspoon onion powder

2 teaspoons sriracha

1 clove garlic, minced

1 teaspoon Dijon mustard

1 tablespoon reduced-sugar ketchup

1 teaspoon Worcestershire sauce

Preheat the oven to 400°F.

In a large bowl, combine the ground beef, breadcrumbs, soy sauce, sriracha, onion, salt, and pepper and form into 8 meatballs.

In a medium bowl, combine the cucumber, rice wine vinegar, and chili flakes (if using). Toss the cucumber so it's well coated and set aside in the refrigerator.

Arrange the meatballs on a baking sheet covered with parchment paper and bake for 10 to 15 minutes until cooked through.

To make the sauce, combine the mayonnaise, onion powder, sriracha, garlic, mustard, ketchup, and Worcestershire sauce in a medium bowl and mix well.

Once the meatballs are cooked, add them to the bowl of sauce and toss until they are well coated. Divide the cooked cauliflower rice and cucumber mixture between two bowls, then divide and add the meatballs.

Serve warm.

LOW-CARB BURGER BOWL

SERVES 2

Burger

½ pound ground beef

¼ teaspoon salt

¼ teaspoon ground black pepper

½ teaspoon garlic powder

⅓ cup shredded cheddar cheese

½ teaspoon Worcestershire sauce

½ teaspoon Dijon mustard

The Bowl

2 cups chopped green lettuce

⅓ cup diced or sliced red onion

½ cup sliced grape tomatoes

1 medium avocado, pitted, peeled, and sliced

½ cup shredded cheddar cheese

2 tablespoons low-carb salad dressing

Add the ground beef to a skillet and cook over medium heat, breaking up the meat with a spatula as it cooks.

Before the meat has cooked through, but when it is no longer pink, add the salt, pepper, and garlic powder and continue cooking. Drain the meat, then reduce the heat to low and add the cheese, Worcestershire sauce, and Dijon, stirring frequently until the cheese melts.

Assemble the two bowls by forming a bed with the lettuce, then topping with the cooked meat, red onion, tomatoes, avocado, and shredded cheese. Drizzle 1 tablespoon of salad dressing on each bowl.

CHICKEN BURRITO BOWL

2 tablespoons extra-virgin olive oil

¼ teaspoon garlic powder

3 tablespoons fresh lime juice

½ teaspoon chili powder

½ teaspoon salt

½ teaspoon cumin

6 ounces boneless, skinless chicken breast

½ cup chopped red bell pepper

2 cups riced cauliflower

½ cup chopped fresh tomato

½ large avocado, peeled, pitted, and cubed

¼ cup grated cheddar cheese

½ cup chopped red onion

¼ cup chopped fresh cilantro

In a small bowl, stir together 1½ teaspoons of the oil, the garlic powder, lime juice, chili powder, salt, and cumin. Add the chicken breast, toss, and let sit in the marinade for 1 to 2 hours.

Remove the chicken from the marinade, place in a skillet, and cook over medium heat until no longer pink inside, about 6 to 8 minutes. When it is done, let cool, then dice it into cubes or small pieces.

Add the chopped pepper and a small amount of the oil to the skillet over medium heat. Cook until tender. Return the chicken to the skillet with the pepper and simmer on low heat.

In another large skillet, add the riced cauliflower and remaining oil and sauté over medium heat while stirring. After a couple of minutes, reduce the heat to low, cover, and simmer for 3 to 5 more minutes. Remove the lid, give the cauliflower a stir, and let the moisture evaporate.

Assemble the two bowls by scooping a cup of cauliflower rice into each bowl, then topping with the chicken, tomato, avocado, cheese, onion, and cilantro. Serve warm.

POKE BOWL

Spicy Mayonnaise Sauce

3 tablespoons mayonnaise

2 teaspoons sesame oil

Juice from half a lemon

2 teaspoons sriracha

The Bowl

6 ounces tuna or salmon, cut into 1-inch cubes

½ cup scallions

¼ cup diced white onion

1 medium cucumber, peeled and diced

½ large avocado, peeled, pitted, and diced

2 tablespoons reduced-sodium soy sauce

3 ounces spring salad mix

⅓ cup chopped walnuts, pecans, or macadamia nuts

1 teaspoon black sesame seeds

To make the sauce, mix the mayonnaise, oil, lemon juice, and sriracha in a small bowl.

In a medium bowl, combine the fish, scallions, onion, cucumber, avocado, and soy sauce. Toss gently, then add the spicy mayo sauce, reserving 1 teaspoon for drizzling at the end.

Break up the spring mix leaves into smaller pieces and divide between two bowls.

Scoop the tossed fish mixture onto the leaves. Top with the nuts and sesame seeds and drizzle with the remaining spicy mayonnaise sauce.

PHILLY CHEESE STEAK BOWL

2 tablespoons avocado oil, plus more as needed

1 small onion, thinly sliced

4 ounces mushrooms, thinly sliced

1 clove garlic, minced

½ green bell pepper, thinly sliced

½ red bell pepper, thinly sliced

One 6-ounce ribeye steak, thinly sliced

Sea salt and black pepper

2 slices of provolone cheese

Add the oil to a large skillet over medium-high heat. Add the onion, mushroom, garlic, and bell peppers and sauté until the mushrooms and peppers are slightly browned and the onion is translucent. Remove from the pan and set aside.

Season the steak slices with salt and pepper. Turn the heat up to medium-high and add a touch of oil to the skillet. Once hot, add the steak. Stir occasionally so as not to burn the steak but to cook it through, about 5 minutes.

Turn the heat down, return the veggies to the skillet, and combine. Divide into two equal portions in the skillet and cover each portion with a slice of provolone cheese. Once the cheese has melted, place a portion of the steak and veggies in each of two bowls. Serve warm.

SNACKS

BACON GUAC BOMBS

2 BOMBS PER SERVING

5 large slices of bacon

1 small avocado

1 clove garlic, crushed

½ teaspoon cumin

¼ cup butter, softened

2 tablespoons chopped
fresh cilantro

2 tablespoons freshly
squeezed lime juice

½ teaspoon crushed chile
pepper

½ small white onion, diced

Kosher salt and freshly
ground black pepper

Preheat the oven to 375°F.

Line a baking sheet with parchment paper and arrange the bacon on the paper, making sure the slices don't touch.

Cook the bacon in the oven until just shy of crispy, but not overcooked. This should take about 10 to 12 minutes. Set the bacon aside.

Cut the avocado in half, remove the pit, and peel. Place the avocado, garlic, cumin, butter, cilantro, lime juice, and chile pepper in a medium bowl and mash well. Add the onion and mix in well. Season with salt and pepper to taste.

Cover the bowl and refrigerate the guacamole for 30 minutes.

Crumble the bacon into small pieces on the baking sheet.

Remove the guacamole from the fridge and form 8 balls, using a spoon. Roll each ball in the bacon bits until well coated. Place the coated balls on a separate tray. Serve at room temperature. (Note: You can refrigerate leftovers to eat later. Store in an airtight container in the fridge for up to a week.)

BACON AVOCADO BOMB

SERVES 2

1 large avocado

½ cup shredded cheddar
  cheese

4 slices of bacon

Preheat the oven to 450°F. Line a baking sheet with parchment paper.

Cut the avocado in half crosswise (not lengthwise), peel, and remove the pit.

Scoop out a small amount of flesh from the center of the avocado to create a bigger well for the cheese.

Fill the avocado wells with cheese, then rejoin the halves. Wrap the avocado with 4 slices of bacon.

Place the bacon-wrapped avocado on the prepared baking sheet and bake for about 5 minutes.

Once the bacon on the top side is cooked through, turn over the avocado, using tongs, and continue baking for another 5 minutes until the other side is cooked.

Remove the avocado from the oven and slice in half to make 2 servings.

BACON-WRAPPED ASPARAGUS BITES

SERVES 2

3 asparagus spears

Extra-virgin olive oil to
  brush the asparagus

2 slices of bacon

Preheat the oven to 450°F. Line a baking sheet with parchment paper.

Wash the asparagus, then trim the bottom of each spear to make it 6 inches long. Cut each spear in half to make 6 three-inch pieces. Brush each piece lightly with olive oil.

Cut the bacon into thirds, then wrap each spear with the bacon and secure the ends with toothpicks.

Place the asparagus on the prepared baking sheet and bake until the bacon is crisp (approximately 10 minutes) or to your desired consistency.

Let cool for a couple of minutes, then serve warm.

LOW-CARB CHOCOLATE CHIP COOKIES

SERVES 7

3 COOKIES PER SERVING

3 cups almond flour

½ cup sweetener of your choice (such as monk fruit, yacón syrup, or stevia)

½ teaspoon baking soda

¼ teaspoon salt

½ cup sugar-free chocolate chips

2 eggs

1 tablespoon pure vanilla extract

¾ cup coconut oil or ½ cup melted butter

Preheat the oven to 350°F. Line a large baking sheet with parchment paper.

In a medium bowl, combine the flour, sweetener, baking soda, salt, and chocolate chips. Mix well.

In a separate bowl, combine the eggs, vanilla, and coconut oil and mix until creamy.

Add the wet ingredients to the dry ingredients and mix with an electric hand mixer or a spoon until the dough is well formed.

Scoop 1-inch balls of dough onto the prepared baking sheet, flatten them slightly, and bake for approximately 10 minutes or until golden brown.

AVOCADO FRIES

4 FRIES PER SERVING

½ cup almond meal

½ cup keto breadcrumbs

½ teaspoon garlic powder

½ teaspoon chili powder

½ teaspoon cumin

½ teaspoon sea salt

2 large eggs

½ cup almond flour

2 large avocados, ripe but firm

Avocado oil spray

Preheat the oven to 425°F. Line a baking sheet with parchment paper and spray with oil.

In a large shallow dish, stir together the almond meal, breadcrumbs, garlic powder, chili powder, cumin, and salt. In a small bowl, beat the eggs. Place the flour in another small bowl. (Note: The bowls need to be big enough to accommodate the avocado slices when you dip them in the coating.)

Remove the pits from the avocados and peel them. Cut each avocado into 8 slices.

Dip each avocado slice in the flour first, making sure it's fully coated and shaking off any excess. Then dip the slice into the egg mixture so that it's fully coated. Finally, dip it in the breadcrumb mixture and shake off any excess.

Place the avocado slices on the prepared baking sheet and lightly spray each slice with oil. Bake for 10 to 15 minutes or until golden brown and crispy. Serve warm or at room temperature.

BURGER FAT BOMBS

2 BOMBS PER SERVING

½ pound ground beef

¼ teaspoon cumin

1½ teaspoons garlic powder

Sea salt and freshly ground black pepper

1 tablespoon cold butter, cut into 10 small pieces

Cheddar cheese, cut into 10 small cubes or 1-inch flat squares

Preheat the oven to 350°F. Lightly grease a mini-muffin tin with cooking spray.

In a small bowl, season the beef with the cumin, garlic powder, salt, and pepper and mix well to distribute seasoning.

Form 10 small flat circles with the beef. Place 1 piece of the butter and 1 square of the cheese on each beef patty, then roll into a ball so that the cheese and butter are completely encased in the middle of the beef ball.

Place the balls in the muffin tin and bake for approximately 15 minutes or until cooked through. Serve warm. (Note: For more fat and flavor, wrap each beef ball with bacon, then bake until the bacon has cooked to your desired doneness.)

COOKIE DOUGH FAT BOMBS

2 BOMBS PER SERVING

½ cup butter, softened

8 ounces cream cheese, room temperature

¼ cup sweetener of your choice (such as monk fruit, yacón syrup, or stevia)

1 cup almond flour

1 teaspoon vanilla extract

⅛ teaspoon salt

½ cup sugar-free chocolate chips

In a large bowl, combine the butter, cream cheese, and sweetener and use an electric hand mixer to beat until fluffy.

Add the flour, vanilla, and salt and mix until combined. Fold in the chocolate chips.

Scoop 1-tablespoon-size balls onto waxed paper. Refrigerate or freeze until hardened to your desire.

MEAT-STUFFED PEPPERS

2 small red bell peppers

1 tablespoon extra-virgin olive oil

½ pound ground beef

1 teaspoon kosher salt

½ small onion, chopped

1 clove garlic, minced

½ teaspoon chili powder

½ teaspoon dried oregano

1 teaspoon brown mustard

¼ teaspoon onion powder

Ground black pepper

1 small plum tomato, diced

Preheat the broiler. Line a roasting pan with aluminum foil. Set oven rack about 8 inches from the heat source if possible.

Cut the tops off the bell peppers and remove the seeds and membranes. Rinse the peppers under cold water.

Bring a large pot of water to boil over high heat. Add the peppers to the pot, reduce the heat, and simmer for 5 minutes or until tender. Drain and set the peppers aside.

In a medium skillet over medium-high heat, heat 1½ teaspoons of the olive oil. Brown the beef, about 15 to 20 minutes. Season with ½ teaspoon of the salt. Remove with a slotted spoon and set aside.

Pour out the excess grease from the skillet and heat it again over medium-high heat. Add the remaining 1½ teaspoons olive oil. Then add the onion and garlic and stir until softened and fragrant, about 2 to 3 minutes. Add the chili powder, oregano, mustard, and onion powder and stir to coat the onion. Season with the remaining ½ teaspoon salt and pepper to taste.

Add the tomato. Stir to combine and simmer for 3 to 4 minutes. Add the meat and simmer until heated through.

Fill the bell peppers with the beef mixture and place them upright in the roasting pan. Broil for 3 to 5 minutes until heated through. Serve warm. (Note: For a snack, eat only one pepper. For lunch or dinner, you can eat two.)

SMOOTHIES

STRAWBERRY DELIGHT SMOOTHIE

SERVES 2

1 cup unsweetened almond milk, coconut milk, or milk of your choice

½ cup full-fat Greek yogurt

1 cup crushed ice

1 cup frozen strawberries, halved

In a high-speed blender, blend the milk, yogurt, and ice until well combined. Add the strawberries and blend until the desired level of creaminess is achieved.

Pour the smoothie into two glasses and enjoy one immediately, saving the other for later.

CREAMY FATTY AVOCADO SMOOTHIE

SERVES 2

1 cup unsweetened
  almond or coconut milk

½ cup full-fat Greek yogurt

½ teaspoon vanilla extract

10 ice cubes

1 large avocado, peeled,
  pitted, and sliced

In a high-speed blender, blend the milk, yogurt, vanilla, and ice until combined.

Add the avocado slices and blend until desired creaminess is achieved. Pour into two cups and enjoy!

MIXED BERRY SUPREME SMOOTHIE

SERVES 2

1 cup unsweetened almond or coconut milk

½ cup full-fat Greek yogurt

1 cup frozen blueberries and strawberries

½ teaspoon vanilla extract

5 ice cubes

In a high-speed blender, blend the milk, yogurt, berries, vanilla, and ice until combined and level of desired creaminess is reached. Pour into two cups and enjoy!

LUSCIOUS CHOCOLATE SMOOTHIE

SERVES 2

1½ cups unsweetened almond or coconut milk

½ avocado, peeled, pitted, and sliced

¼ cup nut butter (such as almond, cashew, or hazelnut)

½ teaspoon vanilla extract

2 tablespoons monk fruit sweetener

10 ice cubes

2 tablespoons unsweetened cocoa powder

In a high-speed blender, blend the milk, avocado, nut butter, vanilla, sweetener, and ice until combined.

Add the cocoa powder and blend until desired creaminess is reached. Pour into two cups and enjoy!

10

SNACKS

Given the popularity of the keto lifestyle, manufacturers are now making popular snacks more keto-friendly and most grocery stores now sell snacks that are labeled "keto" on the packaging. Just because something is labeled keto, however, doesn't give you permission to gorge on it. Remember, with the **Met Flex Diet** plan you are trying not only to improve your metabolic flexibility but also to lose weight. Keeping your snacks to 150 calories or less will go a long way toward preventing you from overeating and packing on pounds instead of shedding them.

The following two lists are by no means comprehensive, but you should have enough options here to find snacks that you like, with plenty of variety. If you want to eat snacks that are not on the list, you are free to do so, but make sure they are 150 calories or less. The snacks are sorted into two lists to make them easier to use: on one list are snacks for keto or low-carb days, and on the other are snacks for those days when you are carb-loading or don't have to follow a more restrictive low-carb regimen. Remember, snacks are meant to be bridges between meals. They are not meals in themselves, so keep that in mind when choosing your portions.

KETO-FRIENDLY

Remember to consume only a quantity that adds up to 150 calories or less.

- Avocado chips
- 2 Burger Fat Bombs (page 208)
- Keto ice cream
- Cheese puffs (keto-friendly)
- Bacon Guac Bombs (page 202)
- Cucumber sushi
- Cookie Dough Fat Bombs (page 209)
- Bacon-Wrapped Asparagus Bites (page 205)
- Low-Carb Chocolate Chip Cookies (page 206)
- 2 hard-boiled eggs
- 10 baby carrot sticks and 2 tablespoons avocado or guacamole dip
- 3 Ham, Cheese, and Egg Rolls (page 147)
- ¾ cup roasted Brussels sprouts
- Bacon Avocado Bomb (page 204)
- Meat-Stuffed Peppers (page 210)
- Keto tortilla chips (100-calorie serving) and 2 tablespoons guacamole
- 8 to 10 zucchini fries
- Keto brownies (150-calorie serving)
- 3 ounces cheddar cheese crisps (prepackaged)
- ½ avocado stuffed with 3 ounces tuna or salmon
- BLT lettuce wrap: 2 slices of bacon, 2 slices of tomato, and 1 tablespoon shredded cheese wrapped in a large romaine lettuce leaf

- 1-ounce bag of kale chips
- ¼ cup cinnamon toasted pumpkin seeds: in a small bowl, combine 1 ounce pumpkin seeds, 1 tablespoon extra-virgin olive oil, and ½ teaspoon cinnamon; spread on a baking sheet and bake at 325°F for 35 minutes
- String cheese (150-calorie serving)
- 3 blue cheese–stuffed apricots: cut apricots in half and remove pits; in a small bowl, mix ⅓ cup blue cheese crumbles, ⅛ teaspoon salt, and 2 teaspoons extra-virgin olive oil; stuff apricot halves with blue cheese mix; place on parchment paper on a baking sheet and bake at 375°F for 2 to 3 minutes
- Beef jerky (no sugar added, 150 calories or less)
- 1 dill pickle wrapped in turkey or ham
- 10 cheese crisps: thinly slice cheddar cheese and place slices on a parchment-lined baking sheet; bake at 375°F until crisp
- 2 tablespoons nut butter (no sugar added) and three 4-inch celery sticks
- Pepperette meat sticks (150-calorie serving)
- 2 cups keto popcorn
- Salmon cucumber bites: spread whipped cream cheese on five cucumber slices; top with small piece of smoked salmon, pepper, salt, and chopped chives
- Caprese salad: cut 2 cups cherry tomatoes in half; add to a medium bowl with 8 ounces mozzarella cubes and ½ cup torn fresh basil leaves; in a small bowl, mix 1 tablespoon balsamic vinegar, 2 tablespoons extra-virgin olive oil, ⅛ teaspoon salt, and ⅛ teaspoon cracked

black pepper; pour oil-vinegar mixture over tomatoes and cheese and toss. (Note: Eat half of the salad and refrigerate the other half and save for later.)

PREPACKAGED KETO-FRIENDLY SNACKS

Many prepackaged keto snacks can be purchased in a store or online. There are too many brands and products to name, but make sure you look for the words "keto," "keto-friendly," or "paleo" on the packaging. Also remember that you're monitoring your snack calorie consumption, so read the labels and make sure you are consuming only 150 calories' worth of the snack. For example, if the nutrition label says 150 calories per serving, but it also says the package contains two servings, then you should consume only half of the package at any one snack time, saving the other half for later.

- Keto chocolate bar
- Beef biltong
- Aged cheddar bar
- Cheddar-flavored almond flour crackers
- Keto peanut butter cookies
- Organic seaweed snacks
- Keto protein bar
- Keto tortilla chips
- Pork rinds (cracklins)
- Smoked bacon bits
- Turkey sticks

- Sweet potato chips
- Almond butter keto cups
- Keto crackers (variety of flavors)
- Keto cups (variety of flavors)
- Keto granola bar
- Protein bark
- Almond butter squeeze pack

FRUIT

The following snacks are 150 calories or less and can be eaten anytime during weeks 1 and 2 and on any of the carb-loading days during the other weeks.

- ½ small apple, sliced, with 2 teaspoons peanut butter
- ¼ cup loosely packed raisins
- 1 cup mixed berries (raspberries, blueberries, blackberries)
- Citrus-berry salad: 1 cup mixed berries (raspberries, strawberries, blueberries, and blackberries) tossed with 1 tablespoon freshly squeezed orange juice
- 2 medium kiwis
- ¼ avocado, smashed, on a whole-grain cracker, sprinkled with balsamic vinegar and sea salt
- Stuffed figs: 2 small dried figs stuffed with 1 tablespoon reduced-fat ricotta and sprinkled with cinnamon
- 1 cup cherries

- 25 grapes
- 1 cup strawberries
- 2 small peaches
- 2 pineapple rings in natural juices
- 2 cups watermelon chunks
- 3 dried apricots stuffed with 1 tablespoon crumbled blue cheese
- Small baked apple (about the size of a tennis ball) dusted with cinnamon
- Chocolate banana: ½ frozen banana dipped in 2 squares melted dark chocolate
- 2 pineapple rounds, each ¼ inch thick, grilled or sautéed
- 5 frozen yogurt-dipped strawberries (dip strawberries in yogurt, then freeze)
- 1 medium grapefruit sprinkled with ½ teaspoon sugar, then broiled if desired
- 6 dried apricots
- 4 dates
- 3 fresh figs
- ½ pound fruit salad
- 1 pomegranate
- 2 small nectarines
- 3 to 4 tablespoons dried cherries
- 1 fat-free mozzarella cheese stick with ½ medium unpeeled apple (about the size of a baseball), sliced
- 1 cup fresh red raspberries with 2 tablespoons plain yogurt

- ½ cup diced cantaloupe topped with ½ cup low-fat cottage cheese
- 1 medium orange, sliced and topped with 2 tablespoons chopped walnuts
- 15 frozen banana slices
- 1 medium mango
- ¾ cup halved strawberries topped with a squirt of whipped cream
- 1 medium papaya with a squeeze of lime juice (sprinkle with chili powder if desired)
- 6 dried figs
- 25 frozen red seedless grapes
- 1 cup raspberries topped with a squirt of whipped cream
- 1 medium apple, sliced, and 1 tablespoon natural peanut butter spread on the slices
- 1 medium pear and 1 cup low-fat or skim milk
- ½ avocado topped with diced tomato and a pinch of pepper
- 1 cup blueberries with a squirt of whipped cream

VEGGIES

- Kale chips: bake ⅔ cup raw kale (stems removed) with 1 teaspoon extra-virgin olive oil at 400°F until crisp
- ½ medium baked potato with a touch of butter or 1 tablespoon sour cream
- 1 medium red pepper, sliced, with 2 tablespoons soft goat cheese

- 10 baby carrots with 2 tablespoons hummus
- 5 cucumber slices topped with ⅓ cup cottage cheese and salt and pepper
- White bean salad: combine ⅓ cup white beans, a squeeze of lemon juice, ¼ cup diced tomato, and 4 cucumber slices
- ⅓ cup wasabi peas
- ½ seeded cucumber stuffed with one thin slice of lean turkey and mustard or fat-free mayonnaise
- Chickpea salad: ¼ cup chickpeas with 1 tablespoon sliced scallions, a squeeze of lemon juice, and ¼ cup diced tomato
- 1 ounce cheddar cheese with 4 to 5 radishes
- 4 to 5 celery sticks with 1 ounce cream cheese
- 2 celery stalks
- 3 oven-baked potato wedges
- 1 large carrot, raw
- ¾ cup carrots, cooked
- 1 cup broccoli florets with 2 tablespoons hummus
- ⅔ cup sugar snap peas and 3 tablespoons hummus
- ½ cup edamame and sea salt to taste
- 1 medium cucumber
- 1 cup lettuce, drizzled with 2 tablespoons fat-free dressing
- Greek tomatoes: chop 1 tomato (about the size of a tennis ball) and mix with 1 tablespoon feta cheese and a squeeze of lemon juice

- Cheesy breaded tomatoes: slice 2 roasted plum tomatoes and top with 2 tablespoons breadcrumbs and a sprinkle of organic Parmesan cheese
- 1 cup sliced zucchini, seasoned with salt to taste
- Grilled portobello mushroom stuffed with roasted veggies and 1 teaspoon shredded low-fat cheese
- 1 cup radishes, sliced or chopped
- 1 medium ear of corn on the cob with seasoning
- 1 medium tomato with a pinch of salt
- ⅓ cup canned red kidney beans
- 1 medium tomato, sliced, with a sprinkle of feta cheese and extra-virgin olive oil
- 1 baked medium tomato sprinkled with 2 teaspoons organic Parmesan cheese
- Black bean salsa over 3 eggplant slices
- 3 medium breadsticks with hummus
- 1 tablespoon peanuts and 2 tablespoons dried cranberries
- 1 cup grape tomatoes
- ¼ cup sliced red bell pepper and ¼ cup thin carrot slices with ¼ cup guacamole
- ½ cup black beans topped with 2 tablespoons guacamole
- Stuffed tomatoes: stuff 10 halved grape tomatoes with a mixture of ¼ cup low-fat ricotta cheese, 1 tablespoon diced black olives, and a pinch of black pepper
- ¾ cup roasted cauliflower with a pinch of sea salt

- 10 baby carrots dipped in 2 tablespoons light salad dressing
- ¾ cup steamed edamame (baby soybeans in the pods)
- ½ medium avocado sprinkled with sea salt
- 1 small baked potato topped with a mixture of salsa and 1 tablespoon shredded low-fat cheddar cheese
- Loaded pepper slices: 1 cup red bell pepper slices topped with ¼ cup warmed black beans and 1 tablespoon guacamole
- 1 medium red bell pepper, sliced, with ¼ cup guacamole
- Tasty pepper: marinate 1 sliced bell pepper in 1 tablespoon balsamic vinegar, and salt and pepper to taste
- ½ cup roasted chickpeas
- 2 dill pickle spears

NUTS AND SEEDS

- 10 to 16 cashews
- 2 tablespoons sunflower seeds
- 17 pecans
- 2 tablespoons poppy seeds
- 2 tablespoons flaxseeds
- 25 peanuts, oil-roasted
- 3 tablespoons roasted, unsalted soy nuts
- 9 to 12 chocolate-covered almonds
- ½ cup shelled pistachios
- ½ cup roasted pumpkin seeds, lightly salted to taste (keep in shells)
- 21 raw almonds

DAIRY

- ½ cup low-fat or fat-free plain Greek yogurt with a dash of cinnamon and 1 teaspoon honey
- 1 small scoop low-fat frozen yogurt
- 2 strips low-fat string cheese
- 1 ounce sharp cheddar cheese cubes
- ½ cup low-fat cottage cheese with ¼ cup fresh pineapple slices
- ½ cup low-fat cottage cheese mixed with 1 tablespoon natural peanut butter
- One 4.5-ounce chocolate fudge sugar-free pudding with 5 sliced strawberries and a squirt of whipped cream
- 1 slice of Swiss cheese and 8 olives
- 2 scoops of sorbet
- ½ cup light natural vanilla ice cream
- 1 cup yogurt parfait and 1 tablespoon granola
- ½ cup no-salt-added cottage cheese and almond butter

PACK-AND-GO SNACKS

- Leaf lettuce roll-up: 1 slice ham or beef and cabbage, carrots, or peppers wrapped in a large lettuce leaf
- Tropical cottage cheese: ½ cup fat-free cottage cheese with ½ cup chopped fresh mango and pineapple
- 1 hard-boiled egg with "everything" bagel seasoning

- 8 to 10 chocolate kisses
- ½ cup fat-free yogurt and ½ cup blueberries
- ½ whole-wheat English muffin topped with 1 teaspoon fruit butter
- 6-ounce glass of orange juice (or frozen juice pops for a cooling treat)
- 2 slices deli turkey breast
- Watermelon salad: sprinkle 1 cup raw spinach and ⅔ cup diced watermelon with 1 tablespoon balsamic vinegar
- Strawberry salad: sprinkle 1 cup raw spinach and ½ cup sliced strawberries with 1 tablespoon balsamic vinegar
- Crunchy kale salad: combine 1 cup chopped kale leaves with 1 teaspoon honey and 1 tablespoon balsamic vinegar
- Cucumber sandwich: top ½ English muffin with 2 tablespoons cottage cheese and 3 slices cucumber
- Cucumber salad: 1 large cucumber, sliced, combined with 2 tablespoons chopped red onion and 2 tablespoons apple cider vinegar
- 1 hard-boiled egg and ½ cup sugar snap peas
- Turkey roll-ups: 4 slices smoked turkey rolled up and dipped in 2 teaspoons honey mustard
- ½ cup unsweetened applesauce with 1 slice whole-wheat toast cut into 4 strips for dunking
- 9 to 10 black olives
- ½ cup Raisin Bran
- 1 cup grape tomatoes and 6 whole-wheat crackers
- 7 saltines

- Spicy black beans: ¼ cup black beans combined with 1 tablespoon salsa and 1 tablespoon fat-free Greek yogurt

- ⅔ ounce dark chocolate

- Mini rice cakes with 2 tablespoons low-fat cottage cheese

- One 11½-ounce can low-sodium V8 100 percent vegetable juice

- ½ sheet matzo

- 20 grapes with 15 peanuts

- ⅓ cup cooked quinoa

- ¼ cup low-fat granola

- ½ cup oat cereal, toasted

- ½ cup clam chowder, preferably tomato-based

- 5 pitted dates stuffed with 5 whole almonds

- ½ cup unsweetened applesauce with 10 pecan halves mixed in

- 4 saltine jelly sandwiches: spread sugar-free jelly between 2 saltine crackers (8 crackers in all)

- Peanut butter and jelly: spread ½ whole-grain English muffin with 1 tablespoon peanut butter and sugar-free jelly

- Egg salad: 1 hard-boiled egg combined with ½ teaspoon low-fat mayo and spices and spread on ½ toasted whole-wheat or whole-grain bagel

- Hummus and cucumbers: chop ½ large cucumber and combine with 2 tablespoons hummus

- Applesauce and cereal: 1 applesauce pouch and ½ cup dry cereal

- 2 hard-boiled eggs with a pinch of salt and pepper

- 2 frozen fruit bars (no sugar added)

- 10 walnut halves and 1 sliced kiwi

- Baby burrito: 6-inch corn tortilla, 2 tablespoons bean dip, and 2 tablespoons salsa

- Kiwi and oats: 1 sliced kiwi with ½ cup oat cereal

- ½ cup natural apple chips (no sugar or preservatives added)

- 2 tablespoons hummus spread on 4 crackers

- 1 cup grapes with 10 almonds

- Chocolate-dipped pretzels: melt semisweet chocolate morsels in a microwave; dip 3 honey pretzel sticks in the chocolate; put the pretzels in the freezer until the chocolate sets

- 50 Goldfish crackers

- 5 pieces of brown rice vegetable sushi rolls

- 1 cup sugar snap peas with 3 tablespoons low-fat hummus

- 1½ cups fresh fruit salad

- ¼ cup yogurt-covered raisins

- 2 celery stalks and 2 tablespoons natural peanut butter

- Watermelon treat: top 1 cup diced watermelon with 2 tablespoons crumbled feta cheese

- 1 cup Cheerios

- 6 watermelon skewers: to make one, place 1 cube of watermelon, 1 small cube of feta cheese, and 1 cucumber slice on a toothpick

- 6 cucumber skewers: to make one, place 1 cucumber slice, a cherry tomato, and a mozzarella ball on a toothpick

- Mediterranean salad: combine 1 sliced tomato; 1 medium cucumber, sliced; and ½ small red onion, diced; then sprinkle with 2 tablespoons low-fat feta cheese
- 1 packet of plain instant oatmeal, ½ cup fresh blueberries, and a sprinkle of cinnamon

MEAT AND SEAFOOD

- 6 large clams
- 3 ounces cooked fresh crab
- 1½ ounces cooked Pacific halibut
- 2 ounces cooked lobster
- 10 cooked bay scallops
- 4 cooked large sea scallops
- 2 ounces cooked yellowfin tuna
- 8 small shrimp and 3 tablespoons cocktail sauce
- 2 ounces smoked salmon
- 6 oysters
- 10 cooked mussels
- ½ cup canned crab
- 3 ounces cooked cod
- 2 ounces lean roast beef
- 4 turkey slices and 1 medium apple, sliced
- 1 can water-packed tuna, drained and seasoned to taste
- 4 ounces chicken breast wrapped in lettuce and topped with dill mustard
- Turkey wrap: 2 slices deli turkey breast, sliced tomato, sliced cucumbers, and lettuce wrapped in whole-grain flatbread

- Turkey-wrapped avocado: ¼ avocado sliced into strips and wrapped in 3 ounces deli turkey meat
- Tuna salad: combine one 5-ounce can water-packed light tuna with 1 tablespoon low-fat mayo and 1 diced sweet pickle

GUILT-FREE TREATS

- 15 mini pretzel sticks with 2 tablespoons fat-free cream cheese
- 25 oyster crackers
- 6 saltine crackers with 2 teaspoons peanut butter
- 4 whole-wheat crackers and 1 ounce fat-free cheese
- 5 tortilla chips and ⅓ cup guacamole
- 1 thin brown rice cake spread with 1 tablespoon peanut butter
- ½-ounce dark chocolate square with 2 teaspoons organic peanut butter
- 3 teaspoons natural peanut butter
- 1 rice cake with 1 tablespoon guacamole
- 3 crackers lightly spread with peanut butter
- 7 animal crackers
- 3 cups air-popped popcorn
- 2 cups air-popped popcorn with 1 teaspoon butter
- 11 blue-corn tortilla chips
- 1½ cups puffed rice
- ½ cup low-fat salsa and 5 small (bite-size) tortilla chips

- 2 graham cracker squares spread with 1 teaspoon peanut butter and sprinkled with cinnamon
- 1 seven-grain Belgian waffle
- 2 Popsicles
- 1 small sliced banana and ½ ounce dark chocolate
- 2 ounces turkey jerky
- English muffin pizza: top 1 whole-wheat English muffin with 1 tablespoon tomato sauce and 1 tablespoon organic Parmesan cheese, then broil
- 2 graham cracker squares and 8 ounces skim milk
- 4 small chocolate chip cookies (each a little larger than a poker chip)
- 10 baked whole-wheat pita chips and 3 tablespoons salsa
- 2 Fudgsicles
- Blueberries and sorbet: ½ cup fruit sorbet topped with ½ cup blueberries
- 1 ounce pretzels and 1 teaspoon honey mustard
- ½ blueberry muffin
- 1 cup strawberries dipped in 1 tablespoon melted semisweet chocolate chips
- 12 small baked tortilla chips and ½ cup salsa
- 7 olives stuffed with 1 tablespoon blue cheese
- 4 potstickers dipped in 2 teaspoons reduced-sodium soy sauce
- 5 crackers lightly smeared with peanut butter
- 2 cups air-popped popcorn sprinkled with 1 tablespoon organic Parmesan cheese

11

EXERCISES

This chapter will help you organize and think about the types of exercises and workouts you want to do while on the program. Obviously, this is not an exhaustive list. There are plenty of other exercises that you can do that will challenge and condition you and help put your body into fat-burning mode. Use this chapter as a resource, but don't feel restricted to it. These exercises are meant to give you food for thought; hopefully you will be inspired to find other exercises as well, or to customize these to meet your needs.

I have divided the exercises into two large categories—traditional cardio exercises and high-intensity interval training (HIIT). You can combine exercises from the two categories to fulfill each day's requirement as spelled out in the **Met Flex Diet** plan. For example, if the day's exercise requirement is a 20-minute, fasted, low-intensity cardio workout, then you would choose from the exercises in the traditional cardio category (or similar exercises). When the plan calls for doing HIIT, then you would choose from the exercises listed in the HIIT category. You will notice that some exercises appear in both categories, according to how you do them. For example, if you ride a stationary or mobile bicycle at a slow pace for a full 10 minutes, that would be a traditional cardio exercise. If you ride the bike in short bursts of intensity followed by periods of rest, that would be HIIT.

I have not included strength and resistance training exercises, which could be an entire book on their own. Don't worry—in just a few seconds, and with a couple of clicks, you can easily find an abundance of these workouts online.

Traditional Cardio

- Cycling (stationary or mobile)
- Elliptical
- Hiking
- Jogging
- Rowing
- Stair climbing
- Swimming
- Walking

HIIT

- Box jumps
- Boxing
- Burpees
- Butt kicks
- Elliptical
- High knees
- Hula hooping
- Ice skaters
- Jumping jacks
- Jump lunges
- Jump rope
- Lunges
- Mountain climbers
- Rowing
- Squat jumps
- Stair climbing

HOW TO PERFORM HIIT

Despite its complex-sounding name, high-intensity interval training is a relatively simple concept. The strategy is to have your body go through short periods of intense energy bursts followed by a period of rest or low-intensity energy output. The beauty of this exercise method is that you can do it with equipment you find in a gym, like an elliptical machine or a treadmill, or you can do it with exercises that don't require gym equipment, like walking or leveraging your own body weight, which is done in calisthenics. Here's what a basic HIIT circuit might look like. You can do this with any of the exercises listed here or with others that are not listed. One of the great features of HIIT is that it's customizable to your preferences, needs, and available resources.

Sample 15-Minute HIIT Circuit

- One cycle: Walk as fast as you can for 30 seconds, then walk slowly for 30 seconds. Do five cycles (repeat five times).

- One cycle: Jump-rope for 30 seconds, then stop and rest for 30 seconds. Do five cycles.

- One cycle: Line-hop for 30 seconds, then stop and rest for 30 seconds. Do five cycles.

The following are some exercises you can do individually, or you can add them to a HIIT routine.

BOX JUMPS

1. Choose a box that fits your physical capabilities, probably between two and three feet high. As your abilities improve, increase the height of the box to create more challenge. Make sure the box can support your weight.

2. Stand in a relaxed position facing the box, knees slightly bent, upper body bent forward on a 45-degree angle, and arms bent back against your sides. This position will help you create momentum.

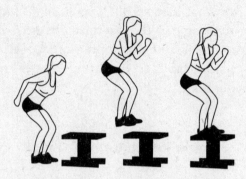

3. In one motion, thrust your arms forward while using your legs to explode into the air and land on the box with both feet in a squat position. Your arms should be in front to help you maintain balance. Don't land on your heels; rather, concentrate on keeping your weight on the balls of your feet.

4. Jump back off the box, returning to the original position, and repeat.

BURPEES

1. Stand with your feet spread hip width apart and your arms resting down by your sides. Lean forward slightly and put more of your weight on the balls of your feet, with your heels slightly off the ground.

2. Lower yourself into a squat position with your knees inside of your hands; steady yourself by placing your hands flat on the floor in front of you.

3. Once you reach the squat position and your hands are on the floor, quickly kick your legs backward, extending your body into a push-up position.

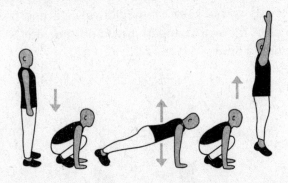

4. Just as you would with a push-up, lower your chest to an inch above the floor, making sure not to touch it.

5. In one motion, push your chest up and kick your legs forward to bring yourself back to a squat position.

6. To complete the burpee, use the power of your legs to push off from the squat position and jump as high as you can straight into the air, with your hands above your head, reaching toward the sky. Start again from step 1.

BUTT KICKS

1. Stand slightly forward, with your feet spread the same width as your shoulders.

2. While moving in a forward direction, kick one foot ahead and the other behind you toward your butt. The hand opposite the foot touching your butt

should simultaneously rise to your shoulder in a pumping motion.

3. As you lift your heels, do not let your thighs move up or down but keep them relatively still and try to do all of the work beneath the knee and with your pumping arms.

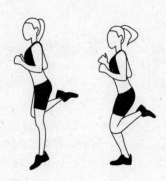

4. It's all right if in the beginning you're not able to touch your butt with your foot. Get it as close as you can. As you become accustomed to the exercise, try to increase your speed and/or duration.

HIGH KNEES

1. Stand erect with your feet apart no wider than your hips. Make sure your arms are hanging down by your sides, with your fists clenched and your back straight, as you look forward.

2. Jump from one foot to the other as if running in place, while lifting your knees as high as you can.

3. Bend your arms 90 degrees and pump them up and down in the same motion as your pumping legs.

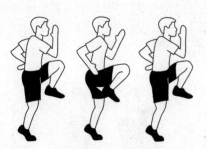

4. Continue the jumping and pumping motion for the duration of the exercise, trying to remain on the balls of your feet and never striking your heels. If you can't do this exercise in full jump mode, you can do a modified, less intense version by marching instead. Using the same motions, pump your arms vigorously and bend your knees as high as you can as you march.

ICE SKATERS

1. Start with your feet placed slightly wider than your shoulders. Looking directly forward, bend your back forward slightly and bend your knees slightly too.

2. In one motion, extend your right leg behind you toward the left side of your body so that it is crossed behind your left leg, then swing your left hand down toward the right side of your body and touch the ground. If you can't bend all the way down and touch the ground, simply swing your left hand to the right side of your body, along your waist.

3. Next, do the same motion on the other side. Bring your right leg back to its starting position and at the same time extend your left leg behind the right side of your body as you touch the ground in front of your left side with your right hand (or swing your right hand along your waist).

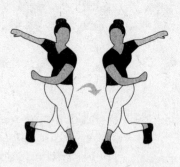

4. Repeat this alternating movement for the desired number of reps.

JUMP LUNGES

1. Start in a lunge position with one leg forward at a 90-degree angle and one leg back, with the knee a few inches above the ground. Make sure you are on the toes of your back foot with the heel off the ground.

2. Bend both arms at the elbow at a 90-degree angle. The arm on the side of the leg that's stretched in front of your body should be reaching forward, and the other arm should be reaching back.

3. Lean forward slightly, tighten your core muscles, then quickly sink your weight down, drive both

feet into the floor, and explode upward in a jump. Extend your knees and hips fully so that you look like a diver jumping on a diving board.

4. While in the air just before landing, switch your arm and foot positions, like a pair of scissors. When you land, the leg and arm that were outstretched before should now be behind you, while the other arm and leg should be in the forward position.

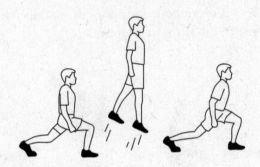

5. To keep your balance and avoid injury, it's important to control your landing. Make sure your forward knee is over your forward foot, not stretched beyond it. Make sure your knees and hips are bent to absorb all of the energy from landing. Be careful to stay flexible around your knees, making sure they aren't locked.

LINE HOPS

1. Stand with both feet together on one side of a line or small object that you can jump over, like a book or a rope. Your hands should be by your sides and bent at a 90-degree angle, as if you are about to run.

2. Crouch down slightly, then explode into the air, jumping up and laterally off both feet at once before clearing the object with both feet at the same time. Land on the other side on the balls of your feet. This is not about jumping as high as you can but about completely clearing the line or object.

3. Once you land, don't rest. Instead, hop right back up and over the object to your original position.

4. Repeat this sequence, continuously jumping from one side to the other without rest.

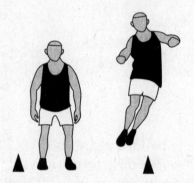

▶ **Modification:** If you have physical limitations and can't jump, don't worry. Rather than jumping over the line, simply place one foot over the line and then quickly bring the other one over, pumping your arms as you do so. Then bring your feet back across the line in reverse order. To get your heart rate up, make sure you do this as fast as you can.

LUNGES

1. Start with your upper body straight and your shoulders held back and relaxed. Keep your chin up, head level, and hands on hips.

2. Engage your core and step forward with one leg by lowering your hips until both knees are at a 90-degree angle—one knee is a step forward bent at a 90-degree angle and the other is bent while almost touching the ground. Keep the knee out front directly above your ankle without pushing it out too far. The other knee should not touch the ground but remain about one to two inches above it.

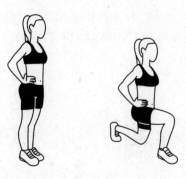

3. Once the lunge is complete, keep the weight in your heels while pushing back up to the starting position.

4. Repeat the sequence, alternating legs.

5. If you want more of a challenge, do the same maneuver, but instead of standing back up to your original position, walk forward doing sequential lunges. This very advanced variation is an excellent way to get your heart rate up and increase your muscle tone.

▶ **Modification:** If you can't independently complete the motions of this exercise, simply use a wall. Face the wall and steady yourself by keeping your hands on it throughout the entire range of motions of the exercise.

MOUNTAIN CLIMBERS

1. Begin in a plank position—hands on the floor, shoulders over your wrists, back straight, body in a downward line, and feet together. You can also rest your forearms on the ground instead of your hands.

2. Keep your upper body still while, in a pumping motion, you bend one leg to bring it forward between your arms and extend the other leg backward. Make sure you maintain your body's line, and don't let your buttocks pop up or your pelvis twist.

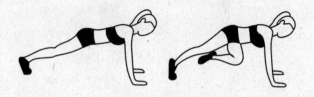

3. Reverse the positions of your legs and repeat. Continue to alternate legs for the duration of the exercise.

SQUAT JUMPS

1. Stand up straight with your feet shoulder width apart and hands by your side.

2. Drop into a squat position with your back bent forward at a 45-degree angle. Bring your arms up together to a 90-degree angle about chest high, with your hands balled into fists or bent into a claw formation. Hold for three seconds.

3. Take a deep breath and then, in one motion, forcefully thrust your arms behind you like a pumping mechanism before exploding into the air, using your hands to help you thrust upward. Land back in the same squat position from which you started.

4. Repeat this sequence for the duration of the exercise.

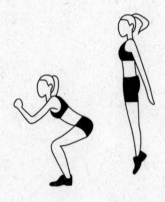

NOTES

1. What Is Metabolic Flexibility?

1. Joana Araújo, Jianwen Cai, and June Stevens, "Prevalence of Optimal Metabolic Health in American Adults: National Health and Nutrition Examination Survey 2009–2016," *Metabolic Syndrome and Related Disorders* 17, no.1 (2019): 46–52, doi:10.1089/met.2018.0105.

2. Improving Your Metabolic Flexibility

1. Gina M. Battaglia, Donghai Zheng, Robert C. Hickner, and Joseph A. Houmard, "Effect of Exercise Training on Metabolic Flexibility in Response to a High-Fat Diet in Obese Individuals," *American Journal of Physiology: Endocrinology and Metabolism* 303, no. 12 (2012): E1440–45, doi:10.1152/ajpendo.00355.2012; Corey A. Rynders, Stephane Blanc, Nathan DeJong, Daniel H. Bessesen, and Audrey Bergouignan, "Sedentary Behaviour Is a Key Determinant of Metabolic Inflexibility," *Journal of Physiology* 596, no. 8 (2018): 1319–30, doi:10.1113/JP273282.

2. Battaglia et al., "Effect of Exercise Training on Metabolic Flexibility in Response to a High-Fat Diet in Obese Individuals."

3. Christophe Kosinski and François R. Jornayvaz, "Effects of Ketogenic Diets on Cardiovascular Risk Factors: Evidence from Animal and Human Studies," *Nutrients* 9, no. 5 (May 19, 2017): 517, doi:10.3390/nu9050517.

4. Harvard T. H. Chan School of Public Health, "The Nutrition Source: Protein," https://www.hsph.harvard.edu/nutritionsource/what-should-you-eat/protein/#protein-research.

6. Week 4: Rhythm

1. Julie E. Flood and Barbara J. Rolls, "Soup Preloads in a Variety of Forms Reduce Meal Energy Intake," *Appetite* 49, no. 3 (2007): 626–34, doi:10.1016/j.appet.2007.04.002.

INDEX

ABOUT THE AUTHOR

Dr. Ian Smith is the author of twenty-three books, including several #1 *New York Times* bestselling books such as *SHRED: The Revolutionary Diet* and *SUPER SHRED: The Big Results Diet*, as well as the bestsellers *Blast the Sugar Out!*, *The Clean 20*, *Clean & Lean*, and *Fast Burn*. He has also authored four novels: *The Blackbird Papers*, *The Ancient Nine*, *The Unspoken*, and *Wolf Point*, three of which have been optioned for film or TV. Dr. Smith is a longtime medical contributor to the Emmy Award–winning *Rachael Ray Show*. He was the solo host of *The Doctors*, the nationally syndicated, Emmy Award–winning television show, and served as the medical/diet expert for six seasons on VH1's highly rated *Celebrity Fit Club*. He was also the creator and founder of the national health initiatives "The 50 Million Pound Challenge" and "The Makeover Mile."

Twitter: DrIanSmith
Instagram: DoctorIanSmith
TikTok: theofficialDrIan
Websites: shredlife.com and doctoriansmith.com